This book is dedicated to the brave and adventurous pioneers in the field of prenatal and infant stimulation, many of whom have made great personal sacrifices for the betterment of the human condition.

It is also dedicated to all the parents who will read this book and wish, as we have many times, if only our parents had done prenatal stimulation before we were born.

# WHILE YOU'RE EXPECTING
## Creating Your Own Prenatal Classroom

by
*F. Rene Van de Carr*, M.D.
and
*Marc Lehrer*, Ph.D

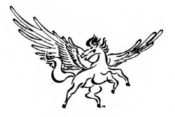

Humanics Trade
P.O. Box 7400
Atlanta, GA 30357

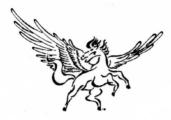

Humanics Trade
P.O. Box 7400
Atlanta, GA 30357

PRINTED IN THE UNITED STATES OF AMERICA

Library of Congress Cataloging-in-Publication Data

Van de Carr, F. Rene
   The prenatal classroom  :  a parents' guide for teaching their preborn baby   /   by F. Rene Van de Carr and Marc Lehrer.
      p. cm.
   ISBN 0-89334-251-3
   I. Prenatal care.          I. Lehrer, Marc.          II. Title.
RG525. V32     1997
618.2'4--dc20

                                                                97-2626
                                                                CIP

Book Design and Illustrations by Susan Chamberlain

# Table of Contents

# Baby's First Kick

Oh, Life, You are there.
A mere imperceptible prod.
That shatters the night
in a time set for nod.

You first spoke to me
without voice;
but so dear.
From my innermost being,
Here
Ma Ma,
I'm here.

**F. Rene Van de Carr, M.D.**

# Editor's Foreword

In December, my wife Jennifer and I found out that we were going to have our first child. In February, I began working on Van de Carr and Lehrer's *Creating Your Own Prenatal Classroom*.

Talk about a take-home assignment.

I had read about the work of the Prenatal Classroom Program in *Omni* and other publications and while I had found their ideas intriguing, it had little to do with my own life. Now here I was, editing their book during the day and coming home to get ready for the baby at night.

In March, Jenny and I began doing some of the Prenatal Classroom exercises and games with our preborn. After I got home from work, we would play the Kick Game and talk, read, and sing to our baby. I would say, "Hi, *baby, this is Da Da,*" and other such odd things with my face on Jenny's abdomen. To our great delight, it worked. After a while, the baby began kicking back where we patted, and in some instances, would even follow the pats around in a circle.

It's hard to describe, but all of a sudden the baby became **real** to me. All the joy, anxiety, and expectation of waiting was tempered by the thought that we were finally going to get to meet this little person with whom we had been playing and talking for all this time.

Elizabeth Hope Hall was born in September. Like any parent, I would be the first to tell you about how exceptional she is, and the advanced age at which she began doing all the things that are, (according to the two dozen or so baby books that all new parents seem to acquire), supposed to come later on in her first year. But that would be missing the point of what I now believe to be one of the main benefits parents, children, and other family members gain by using the Prenatal Classroom program. We established a loving relationship with our baby before she was born. Elizabeth's birth wasn't the beginning of our association, it was more like meeting someone face to face with whom you had only spoken on the telephone. Whatever advances, neurological, lingual, or musical that she might have made in the womb, the fact that her parents love her and are aware of their roles as her first teachers gives her the best advantage a child can have.

When I am older, and think back on the first time I met my daughter, it won't be a delivery room or hospital nursery that will come to mind. Because of the Prenatal Classroom program, it will be a darkened, candle-lit room at home, and the tiny thrust of a kick beneath my hand.

**Robert Hall**

# Acknowledgments

Books are not written by a single person but by a group of people, each contributing his or her expertise to the project. Such was the case with *While You're Expecting: Creating Your Own Prenatal Classroom*. The authors wish to thank the following people for their contributions:

**Kristin Van de Carr**, Ph.D, Dr. Van de Carr's wife, and a researcher and international lecturer whose work in prenatal psychology has been one of the cornerstones of this book.

**Leslie Lehrer**, Dr. Lehrer's wife who housed and birthed two wonderful children, Celene Lora and Claire Jenevieve.

**Sharon L. Van de Carr**, who turned a collection of exercises, research, anecdotes, and theories into a comprehensive manual.

**Cathy Guisewite**, famed cartoonist who brought additional national attention to The Prenatal University through her comic strip "Cathy."

# Author's Preface to the First Edition

The Prenatal Classroom program came out of the pioneering work on prenatal education first developed in 1979 by Dr. Rene Van de Carr, an obstetrician based in Hayward, California. The program was initially called the Prenatal University and has been gradually developed and expanded into the comprehensive Prenatal Classroom program for preborns, newborns, and family members.

Dr. Marc Lehrer, a psychologist formerly with the Child Study Unit at the University of California Medical School in San Francisco, joined Dr. Van de Carr in developing additional prenatal stimulation and bonding exercises. Together they investigated the effects of prenatal stimulation on the growing number of youngsters whose parents had used Dr. Van de Carr's exercises.

The goal of the Prenatal Classroom program is to help parents and family members foster a better fetal environment for the baby, provide opportunities for early learning enhancement, and promote the development of a positive relationship between parent and child that can last a lifetime.

We have been collecting data on the more than 3,000 children who have been through the Prenatal University program in Hayward, California. We have published scientific articles about these children and have given numerous lectures, conferences, and interviews on national television and for domestic and international magazines.

Some humorous elements of the program have even found their way into a daily newspaper comic strip called "Cathy," by Cathy Guisewite, who obtained information from the doctors in preparing her story line.

This and many other forms of worldwide publicity have made some of the basic ideas of the Prenatal Classroom available throughout the United States and many other countries. Unfortunately, most of the television spots and even the full-length magazine articles barely touch upon the practical ways to teach your baby before birth.

Most coverage continues to emphasize having "smarter" babies but rarely discusses the incredible good feelings and positive bonding that can occur among family members who use our program before the baby is born. In response to numerous inquiries for more information, we decided to publish the materials we use in the Prenatal Classroom program. We hope you will join the many thousands of satisfied families who have used our program.

cathy®     by Cathy Guisewite

IT'S TYPICAL FOR WOMEN WHO HAVE BEEN REAL GO-GETTERS IN BUSINESS TO TURN THAT SAME PASSION ONTO THE EXPERIENCE OF PARENTING.

SOME START WITH FLASH CARDS AND MUSIC LESSONS WHEN THEIR BABY IS JUST A WEEK OLD. YOU'RE NOT GOING TO DO THAT ARE YOU, ANDREA?

START EDUCATING THE BABY A WEEK AFTER BIRTH?? DON'T BE RIDICULOUS.

WE WOULD HAVE MISSED THE WHOLE NINE MONTHS OF PREGNANCY!

..THIS NEXT SELECTION IS FROM VIVALDI, LITTLE ONE...

## Using the Term "Preborn" Rather Than "Fetus"

*Fetus* is a technical and medical term that most often has been applied to the physical development of the baby prior to birth. Our work is concerned more with enhancing the physical and mental capabilities of the baby prior to birth and in helping to create better mother, father, and familial bonding with the baby before birth. *Preborn* refers to physical, mental, and emotional stages of development in the baby before birth in the same way that newborn, infant, and toddler refer to specific developmental progressions after birth. For this reason, we believe that the term *preborn* best respects the developing awareness of the baby you carry throughout your pregnancy.

## What You Will Learn

The first section of this book answers your questions about the Prenatal Classroom. The second section provides a guide to proper nutrition and activity for a healthy pregnancy. The third section, the heart of Prenatal Classroom, teaches communication between yourself and your preborn baby. The final section shows you how to continue those methods with your newborn. We also have our own post-birth program for stimulating your baby, but the Prenatal Classroom curriculum can easily interface with post-birth programs developed by others in this field.

The Prenatal Classroom program shows you a practical, everyday way of teaching your baby before he or she is born. These same exercises and methods can be applied during the months after your baby is born even if you didn't use the program before birth. We will provide guidelines for recommended times throughout the day when certain exercises seem to be most beneficial.

All of the recommended learning games have been developed from both of our experiences in explaining the concepts and methods of prenatal stimulation to thousands of families who are expecting a baby and then getting to know their newborn. Even though the exercises are designed for the developing baby, each one also teaches something to the parents about how their baby feels, reacts, and learns.

The Prenatal Classroom also helps participating family members develop positive relationships with the new baby. We believe the intimate awareness that results when establishing a relationship with your baby before it is born can further emotional bonding in the family and promote a deeper appreciation of the miracle of life.

## Who can use the Prenatal Classroom Program?

If you are pregnant, planning to have a baby in the near future, have just had a baby, or have a family member or close friend who is expecting a baby, the Prenatal Classroom Program is for you. You can use and enjoy many of the principles and some of the exercises with your newborn even if you didn't use the program during pregnancy or had a late start.

## What about Skeptics of Prenatal Stimulation?

For more than eight years we have presented information about our program at international conferences and professional meetings, in professional journal and magazine articles and on numerous national and international television programs. We have enjoyed overwhelming support from parents who tried at least some of our methods or who had discovered them on their own and wrote to tell us. As has been the case with any new approach to childrearing, there are adherents and detractors. There will always be critics of any innovative program.

While it is nice to have the acclaim of the media and our professional colleagues, we have looked to our Prenatal Classroom participants (the people who have actually had the babies and raised the children) to make the final determination about the value of our program. What we do makes sense to many parents. Furthermore, we believe that in many cases mothers, fathers, and grandparents have already been doing many of the exercises that we advocate such as singing to their baby and patting when the baby kicks, throughout the history of humanity.

What we have done is systematized prenatal stimulation exercises so you can pick and choose a set of exercises that makes sense to you. We have also included guidelines for nutrition and birthing that fit with the most up-to-date, scientific understandings of prenatal stimulation practices.

We believe that everyone, the developing baby included, has a right to an education. Children can eventually learn to read a little by themselves, but isn't it easier to learn if a caring teacher goes over vowel sounds and alphabet recognition skills with them? In the same way, when you are consistent in using the Prenatal Classroom exercises, your baby has an opportunity to learn what otherwise might be forever lost.

**F. Rene Van de Carr, M.D.**
**Marc Lehrer, Ph.D.**

# Author's Preface to the Second Edition

The Prenatal Classroom was first published in 1992 and represented our efforts to document the prenatal program that Dr. Rene Van De Carr had first developed in 1979. The program had progressively become more comprehensive and had received much national and international publicity throughout the 1980's and into the 1990's. Our work was being referred to in books, articles, and on radio and television shows based upon the manuals, video tapes and audio tapes we had created and sent to all eager parents and to prenatal programs throughout the United States and in many other countries as well. Several countries including Venezuela and Thailand had created prenatal education programs modeled after our work and based on our consultations with heads of their programs.

Talking with and playing music to your baby before birth has started to become something many parents to be were doing, worldwide. Most mothers got the idea from television shows or magazine articles that doing these activities with their yet to be born child seemed like something good to do, and also might be easy and fun. Even more significantly, their doctors and other health care providers involved with prenatal care, when asked by their patients, seemed supportive their using prenatal stimulation methods. What a change from those times in the early 1980's when almost no physicians admitted that babies had any degree of awareness or ability to learn in the first months following birth, let alone during the prenatal period. The long road of our efforts to help convince the public to use these methods has finally come to fruition.

Yet most parent to be only had a few bits and pieces of the information used in the comprehensive program of prenatal stimulation we had developed. With the publication of the first edition of this book, *The Prenatal Classroom*, we felt we had finally made available a full version of the program for those who wanted to use it and perhaps our job was done.

Here it is four years later, 16 years after the first of many thousands of patients had begun to use the program. And now a new edition, why?

First, and foremost, new research and replication of previous preliminary research has continued to show what we had maintained all along, that these methods work. They help babies develop more intelligence and self assurance that remains with them as they grow and thrive. Furthermore, they communicate better with their parents and other family members. Finally, they have greater self confidence than their peers.

Here are some of the significant new findings and developments that have come about since the publication of the first edition of the Prenatal Classroom:

**A)** The American Association of the Advancement of Science in 1996 summarized the work of a number of researchers in prenatal and infant stimulation.

**1)** Dr. Craig Ramey at the University of Alabama showed that early stimulation programs increased intelligence test scoring in all children followed from early infancy to the 15th year in a major study. Children attained 15 to 30 percent higher intelligence scores.

**2)** Dr. Marion Cleves Diamond of the University of California at Berkeley, experimenting over many years and replicating results numerous times, has shown that stimulated rats not only developed more brain cell branching and thicker cortical areas of the brain, but they also were "smarter" and were more socially skilled in their behaviors with other rats.

**3)** Dr. Hugo Moser at Johns Hopkins University has reported work with Rhesus Monkeys that were stimulation deprived. This resulted in striking and distressing defects in their behavior as they matured. They became clumsy, self abusive and withdrawn from social contact with other monkeys and showed every sign of limited intelligence.

**B)** The Prenatal Enrichment Unit at HuaCchiew General Hospital in Bangkok Thailand under the direction of Dr. C. Panthuraamphorn has now replicated our findings originally published in the mid 1980's showing that prenatally stimulated babies have early acquisition of speech, early imitation of speech sounds, earlier first word, early spontaneous smiling, earlier turning of their heads toward the sounds of their parents' voices, respond better to music and also develop better social patterns as they mature. Dr. Panthuraamphorn first visited our programs in 1989 and set up his programs based upon our consultations. It is most heartening to see how he has attained the same results we reported on in a totally different environment and culture using controlled studies.

**C)** Dr. Beatriz Manrique, President of CEDIHAC (The Venezuela Ministry For the Development of Intelligence) has now reported results of over 600 babies who were pre and post natally stimulated and followed initially over a three year period. These babies, in comparison to their non-stimulated peers, were most "oriented", had better acceptance of breast feeding, showing they and their mothers were more comfortable with each other; had better language development; better hand-eye coordination; better problem solving abilities and fewer instances of developmental delay (which was especially significant since these studies were conducted with very poor social economic populations). Dr. Manrique has concluded in her most recent articles that the youngsters who received stimulation and have now been followed up to 6 years have continued to increase their intelligence scores and are thus widening the intelligence gap, leaving their non stimulated peers further and further behind.

Shouldn't everybody be using prenatal stimulation with their preborns? We think so. Let's give our babies the best chance to deal with the every increasing complex world to which we have brought them. They deserve it.

**Rene F. Van de Carr, M.D.**
**Marc Lehrer, Ph.D.**

# WHILE YOU'RE EXPECTING
*Creating Your Own Prenatal Classroom*

# PART I
## *Parents' Questions*

## *Can my preborn baby really learn?*

Our own research and that of innumerable scientists in the field of prenatal development has shown that inside the uterus the baby is capable of learning, feeling, and telling the difference between dark and light. By the time you are five months (20 weeks) pregnant, your baby's ability to "sense" stimuli has sufficiently developed for you to begin playing learning games.

Your first job is to get baby's attention. In doing so, it may be helpful to consider the fact that people who live near a freeway seldom notice the noise of the cars going by. In a similar way, the baby inside your womb hears noises and feels vibrations and movement. But because these stimuli have no meaning or pattern, the baby cannot learn from them and tends to ignore sounds and motions outside of his environment.

For example, we have had a number of parents tell us how their babies responded after birth to music they heard before birth. A well-known example of this phenomenon was reported by our colleague, Dr. Thomas Verny in his book, *The Secret Life of the Unborn Child*. Dr. Verny wrote about an interview in which famed symphony conductor Boris Brott discussed how he had become interested in music. The conductor remembered that as a young man he found he had the ability to play certain pieces of music without practice:

*I'd be conducting a score for the first time and suddenly the cello line would jump out at me. I'd know the flow of the piece before I found the page on the score. One day I mentioned this to my mother, who is a professional cellist. I thought she would be intrigued because it was always the cello line that was so distinct in my mind. She was very intrigued, but when she heard what the pieces were, the mystery solved itself. All the scores I knew by sight were the ones she had played while she was pregnant with me.*

We believe the kind of sounds generated by the cello that provided Brott's early stimulation are quite significant. The sounds of the cello are not too loud, they vibrate through the air, and the cello is played by holding it close to the womb where both the sounds and vibrations can be clearly felt as well as heard.

When the mother was pleased with her performance, this biological message of pleasure would be transmitted to the baby. The baby would associate the sound of the music with the biochemical message of pleasure. Biological messages can also be sent from mother to baby if mother is a smoker (see page 25).

Our program includes structured exercises which help teach your baby in a similar manner. However, we do not require that parents learn to play the cello or any other difficult instrument in order to do these exercises. Instead, we suggest you use a small drum. How and when will be explained in a later chapter.

## How do I communicate with my baby?

Many parents ask us what we mean by communication with a pre-born baby. The easiest way to explain this is for you to think about how your own senses are affected when you are talking with someone you know well and care about. Communication is a lot more than passive listening: you hear a voice, you feel a touch, you see an image, and you feel an emotion. They are all part of the communication process.

Similarly, your preborn baby is capable of learning to pay attention to the sounds of your voice (and your husband's, other children's, grandparents', etc.) or music, touches through your abdomen, changes from light to dark, and even Mommy's emotions. In some circumstances, he or she may respond with a kick or other movement.

In the Prenatal Classroom program we have you begin the process of communication with exercises that are similar to what most parents already do. For example, many mothers naturally pat back when baby begins to kick during the fifth month of pregnancy. Mothers have also rocked to music, sung to their babies, and read stories to them during pregnancy. We have taken the best methods suggested to us by parents, modified others, and created entirely new ones for you to communicate with your baby before birth.

We teach you how to continue these actions after birth as a game that is helpful for the baby's developing cognitive abilities. Words that can be associated with certain sounds or sensations are also used to stimulate the preborn baby. This is done by showing you how to communicate with the baby using touch, vibration, motion, sound, and light.

*My husband and I had a fight the other day. He and I were both yelling our heads off. The baby started kicking me harder and harder so I finally had to sit down because it hurt. So the baby really stopped the fight.*

(Pregnant mother in her eighth month talking with Dr. Van de Carr)

2

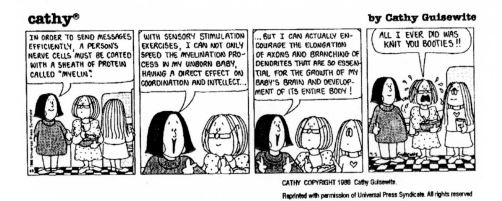

cathy®                                    by Cathy Guisewite

**Panel 1:** IN ORDER TO SEND MESSAGES EFFICIENTLY, A PERSON'S NERVE CELLS MUST BE COATED WITH A SHEATH OF PROTEIN CALLED "MYELIN".

**Panel 2:** WITH SENSORY STIMULATION EXERCISES, I CAN NOT ONLY SPEED THE MYELINATION PROCESS IN MY UNBORN BABY, HAVING A DIRECT EFFECT ON COORDINATION AND INTELLECT...

**Panel 3:** ...BUT I CAN ACTUALLY ENCOURAGE THE ELONGATION OF AXONS AND BRANCHING OF DENDRITES THAT ARE SO ESSENTIAL FOR THE GROWTH OF MY BABY'S BRAIN AND DEVELOPMENT OF ITS ENTIRE BODY !

**Panel 4:** ALL I EVER DID WAS KNIT YOU BOOTIES !!

# Are babies who have had prenatal stimulation smarter?

Our colleague, Dr. Marion Diamond of the University of California at Berkeley, did a postmortem analysis of Einstein's brain. Her results showed that Einstein had a greater number of cell structures than is usual in the area of the brain that controls how thoughts are processed. While there is no evidence that Mrs. Einstein practiced prenatal stimulation with young Albert, Dr. Diamond feels that the greater brain growth she likewise finds in prenatally stimulated research animals can be accounted for by the effect on the developing baby of an active and healthy mother. Hormones that stimulate a baby's brain appear to cross the placenta more easily when the mother is active, healthy, and in a stimulating environment.

For example, Dr. Diamond found greater brain growth occurred in prenatally stimulated laboratory rats. One group of pregnant lab rats were kept in their normal, non-stimulating environment. Another group of pregnant lab rats were placed in a stimulating environment with lights, sounds, mazes, and toys to play with. After the rats gave birth to their litters, the offspring of the stimulated rats outperformed the offspring of the non-stimulated rats in mazes and many other tests. Analysis of the brain matter of offspring rats from both groups showed greater brain growth in those rats whose mothers had been stimulated. Diamond's research indicates that even indirect stimulation of developing baby rats through stimulation of their mothers seems to increase their brain growth. We believe Dr. Diamond's findings also hold true with human babies in the womb, which is another reason why we advocate interactive stimulation sessions appropriate for each stage of physical development.

Before birth, it is a regular occurrence in fetal development for a great many nerve cells in baby's brain to die off. Prenatal stimulation gives the brain an opportunity to make use of more brain cells before birth, thus giving the baby a greater total brain capacity and a true "head start" in life.

## How can prenatal stimulation affect a baby's mental growth?

Our research shows the following points in pre-birth stimulated infants:

**1)** There appears to be a critical time in an infant's development beginning at about five months before birth and extending to about two years of life when brain stimulation and intellectual exercise can improve your baby's mental capabilities.

**2)** Prenatal stimulation helps develop your baby's orientation and effectiveness in dealing with the world outside after birth.

**3)** Babies who have received prenatal stimulation may be more in control of their movements and may be better prepared to explore and learn about their environments after birth.

**4)** Parents who have participated in the Prenatal Classroom program have described their babies as more calm, alert, and happy.

In our experience and in the experience of many other professionals in hospitals, clinics, and birth centers, pre-birth stimulated babies are typically more attentive, (especially to their parents' voices) and are more motivated to learn. This results from your having talked to your baby for several months before birth. The baby learns to recognize certain voice patterns as having something to do with his actions. It is then more likely that the baby will be attentive to what you say after birth because he wants to listen to you and the pure, pleasurable sound of your voice, even long before he can fully understand the meaning of your words. You may be able to maintain his or her interest and attention for longer periods of time than is usual. As Prenatal Classroom babies grow, parents report they are good listeners and follow directions well.

Even the birth experience can be made less frightening for the baby. Because the baby comes to know your touch and voice – along with favorite music – before birth, he or she can be reassured by the presence of these familiar sounds and stimulations during delivery. Many fathers report that immediately after birth their babies responded to their voices by turning and looking at them. In each case, the baby, only minutes after birth, was selectively responsive to the father's voice even though there were other men talking in the delivery room.

Many parents of Prenatal Classroom babies have told us that giving their full attention to the baby during stimulation sessions, even for two minutes or less, taught them an important lesson, i.e., these sessions readied them for and helped them feel good about responding to their baby's needs after the birth. Communication is a two-way process. While your baby is learning about you, you are learning about your baby, to everyone's benefit.

## Will our baby really learn the Primary Words and other exercises in this book?

Part of the Prenatal Classroom program consists of familiarizing the baby with a short list of Primary Words before birth. A lot of people have asked if we really believe babies in utero are learning the Primary Words. Our answer is yes, but not in the same way you do.

A preborn baby does not learn as an adult does. When you learn a word, you can repeat it, recognize it in writing as well as in speech, modify it to maintain proper speech (such as changing from the singular to the plural form), and use it in a sentence. Your own thought processes demonstrate to you that you have learned the word.

Your baby is learning in a much more rudimentary way. When you are teaching the Primary Words to your baby, she is hearing those sounds at the same time she is experiencing specific sensations. For example, when you say the word *"pat,"* baby hears the *"p,"* short *"a,"* and *"t"* sounds while you are patting your abdomen. This pairing of sound and experience gives your baby a chance to form connections about sound and sensation at a preverbal level of recognition. You are providing your baby with a head start that cannot be gained any other way.

Over the years we have had a number of reports of very advanced developmental and cognitive abilities from parents who have used these exercises with their babies before birth. We have culled from these reports several findings. Prenatal Classroom babies tend to lift their heads, roll over, sit up, talk, and stand up at an earlier age than their non-stimulated peers. As tiny infants, they move their eyes to look for their parents when they hear their voices. Throughout their infancy and childhood, prenatally stimulated youngsters are less bothered by pain and are seen by their parents as more confident and self assured than other children.

This is true even in the same families when the Prenatal Classroom exercises were used with the second or later children. These parents often tell us the child who received prenatal stimulation developed faster and often spoke earlier than the firstborn, non-stimulated child. We have been following a number of our graduates for more than ten years and are pleased to report that these gains continue.

We believe this is an appropriate time to caution you against becoming unhealthily obsessed or over-involved with "how much" your baby is learning. On one hand, the prenatal education of your baby is secondary to the bonding that is going on between you and your baby, and also between you and your partner and family. On the other hand, the Prenatal Classroom provides some of the most profound and unique educational experiences of a person's lifetime. After all, most people don't remember their first attempts at standing or the first time they said two words together. Yet most parents recall the incredible look on their children's faces when these events occurred. One of our program's original intentions is to provide the opportunity for the same wonderful experiences and memories to be established even before birth. It is our great hope that parents and family members have fun with the exercises. By relaxing, having fun, and learning about your baby while he or she learns about you, the rewards of prenatal stimulation can extend to everyone and endure for a lifetime.

## Will I *expect too much of my baby after birth*? Is prenatal *stimulation going too far too fast*?

Your expectations toward your preborn child count. In 1968, an experiment conducted by Dr. Robert Rosenthal and Dr. Lenore F. Jacobson at an elementary school in South San Francisco Unified School District showed that when a group of teachers who were unfamiliar with the school's population were told a group of good students were poor students, the children received lowered evaluations and performed poorly. Similarly, when teachers were told that poor students were good students, the students' work improved.

Parents who use our program expect their children will pay attention to them and will want to learn. Even if our program did nothing more than raise the parents' expectations to the point where they believe their children can be successful learners, we would think it an overwhelming success.

## Isn't prenatal stimulation unnatural?

On the contrary, prenatal stimulation is one of humankind's oldest and most natural processes.

The story of humanity is filled with instances of ritualistic prenatal stimulation. In so-called primitive societies, pregnancy and birth are often celebrated with ritualized movement, music, and song. There are cultures in which women dance and sing repetitive chants throughout their pregnancy. Some cultures have special chants and ritual assurances for mother and child at birth as well. It is our society that has lost touch with providing active experiences and sensations for the developing baby as an integral part of the overall pregnancy experience. Our lives are often too complex and have few, if any, consistent experiences that might naturally provide what we teach in the Prenatal Classroom.

It may be helpful for you to think of the exercises you do in the Prenatal Classroom as reminders of a rich cultural lore humanity abandoned long ago for a more comfortable, yet mechanized and impersonal society.

## Is it safe to use prenatal stimulations?

Exercises used in the Prenatal Classroom program were developed for use by healthy women with normal pregnancies, and thousands of these women have used the program without any problems. All of the exercises are similar to everyday activities or movements you might perform during pregnancy or involve other stimulation you and your baby might hear, feel, or see during pregnancy. With our program you teach your baby, using sensations by presenting them in systematic ways so that they become learning exercises.

We recommend that every mother using the program advise her doctor, midwife, or birth educator that she is doing so. If you have a specific medical condition that can affect your pregnancy or if you become sick or develop any complication, you should discontinue any exercises or practices until you have had a chance to ask your doctor's advice and continue only with his or her approval.

Although we have seen the many positive-only effects of prenatal stimulation upon the developing baby, we have also become very sensitive to the possibility that negative prenatal stimulation can also occur. It is, of course, possible to overstimulate your preborn baby in the same way you can overstimulate a newborn, a toddler, or a young child. That is why we recommend brief sessions for prenatal stimulation exercises.

Either parent can unwittingly engage in behaviors that can injure their developing babies. Such behaviors include drinking alcohol, smoking, using drugs, not maintaining a nutritionally sound diet, fighting, or participating in an activity in which they may become seriously injured.

Demanding physical activities such as skiing or sky diving can be dangerous to the health of a developing baby, but the baby has no choice other than to participate along with its mother during pregnancy. Can you imagine the degree of overstimulation for the babies of two pregnant women who are professional wrestlers? Or the mental state (passed along to the unborn child) of a mother whose husband drinks to excess, smokes, and verbally or physically abuses his wife? You, as a parent have the ultimate responsibility as to exactly what kind of stimulation, nurturing or otherwise, the baby receives. As always, use good judgment in your choice of activities.

## Is stimulation also useful for premature babies?

We believe parents can apply many of the same Prenatal Classroom exercises and principles with premature infants, as long as the infant seems comfortable with the exercises. Because there are often medical considerations when dealing with premature infants, you should check with your doctor about using the Prenatal Classroom program with your "preemie."

One hospital on the East Coast uses a vibrating electric toothbrush with cotton wrapped around the bristles to give gentle tactile stimulations to premature infants. Another of our colleagues and a collaborating researcher on Prenatal Classroom techniques, Dr. Elvidina Adamson-Macedo of Sterling, England, has been using massage on 32 to 34 week old premature infants, a technique similar to some of the primary sensory experiences (pat, rub, stroke, and squeeze) we discuss in the Primary Word List section.

A recent study by Dr. Ruth T. Gross of the Infant Health and Development Program at Stanford University showed that when premature infants were involved in early stimulation games at home, three years later they scored over 13 points higher on intelligence measures than their peers, who as premature infants had not received stimulation. This study involved 985 infants and was the largest study of its kind.

*The results of this study indicate the effectiveness of a comprehensive intervention, even for biologically vulnerable infants. Our findings show that children who received the intervention (stimulation), experienced significantly higher IQ scores, significantly fewer maternally reported behavior problems.*

(Journal of the American Medical Association, 1990)

Parents in the study seemed to benefit from the games as well. Those who used stimulation learned to be more interactive with their infants. The mothers who stimulated their premature infants were also more alert to their babies' physical conditions.

The results of these studies can be directly related to the gains your developing baby can make through prenatal stimulation. In terms of their development, the only difference between the 7 month old baby in your womb and the 7 month old premature baby is location.

## Who are the teachers in the Prenatal Classroom?

Mother, of course, is baby's primary teacher. Mother's helper will usually be Dad, but it can also be an older child, relative or friend who will be there with you and the baby during pregnancy and after the birth.

Engaging the whole family in these stimulation sessions produces several positive results. First, it promotes togetherness and a sense that every family member, even the youngest, can contribute to baby's education. Second, performing these exercises actually trains family members to be better teachers. Most importantly, the exercises allow each family member to bond with the baby before it is born. This is especially important for siblings who may feel displaced by the new baby. Even your pet can help "teach" baby in the Prenatal Classroom as these comments from some of our mothers attest:

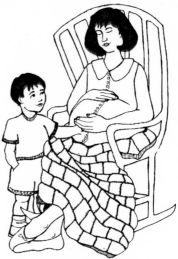

*I think the baby laughs when I do because when my head is on Mommy's tummy and I'm playing with the baby, it kicks my ear.*

(A 6 year old boy discussing how he plays with his preborn sister.)

*My baby really likes it when I put the cat on my stomach! Kitty has a real loud purr, and the baby sort of gently rolls around as long as the cat is there.*

(A Prenatal Classroom mother who noticed the bond between her preborn baby and the family pet. After birth the baby and cat were very good friends even when she pulled the kitty's tail.)

*The baby seems to know when I put my parakeet on my abdomen. It tweets, and the baby moves.*

(Another Prenatal Classroom mother whose pet took part in the exercise.)

## Will I have enough time to do these exercises?

Being a teacher in the Prenatal Classroom is not the full-time job you might think it is. In fact, it doesn't have to take much time at all.

You will be able to play the learning games even if you are working outside your home throughout pregnancy. Some exercises can easily be done at work. One mother used to tell her baby when she was going to lunch, and the baby would move in response.

We suggest two stimulation sessions per day. Our research and more than fifteen years of practical experience with more than 3,000 Prenatal Classroom parents show that only five to ten minutes per session seems to be the ideal schedule for parents and baby.

To make the experience of communicating with your preborn baby a pleasant one, set the sessions aside as special times each day. Create an atmosphere of trust between you, your helpers and baby, and try not to do too much at one time. Setting aside "special times" and creating such an atmosphere with your baby before his or her birth is the basis for the activities we recommend in the Prenatal Classroom.

If possible, set aside time in the morning for one session, which you do alone, and another one in the evening with Dad or another helper participating. Keep in mind that the time of day you choose to stimulate your baby may establish a pattern that carries into his or her life after birth. (For some of the exercises or learning games we will give you specific instructions about the best time to practice.)

*The only time my husband was able to share talking to the baby with me was late at night just before he went to work. Now that Bobby is 3 months old he wakes us at the same time that we were talking to him before he was born. And he won't go back to sleep until he gets a few words from his Dad.*

(Comments from the mother of one of Prenatal University's earliest graduates.)

After hearing comments like this for about a year, we decided to include guidelines for scheduling sessions so your baby is likely to go to sleep and awaken at convenient hours.

Remember, just like you, your preborn baby can get tired. For this reason we do not advocate sessions that last more than ten minutes or that you try to make up for missed teaching time. By the same token, spending twice as much time stimulating your baby will *not* be twice as good for his or her developing intelligence. In fact, some studies show too much stimulation tires infants and may even prevent learning. Therefore, keep your sessions short.

It is most important that you, the parent-teacher, recognize the exercises are to be used in very special ways with your baby. We are not trying to force learning upon the baby. Again, the exercises are meant to be fun for you, your baby, and your helpers. If the exercises are done in this way, then in addition to your baby learning, you will learn some very importat principles of relating to your child after he or she is born.

## What can I learn from the Prenatal Classroom exercises?

**1)** If you give your full attention to your baby even before he or she is born, you are likely to get back a good response.

**2)** By focusing your full attention on your baby before birth, you are developing a good habit of relating to him or her that can last a lifetime. It is often easier to do this before the distractions of parenthood steal away your concentration.

**3)** Involving Dad and brothers and sisters as helpers in stimulation sessions will help them relate to baby after he or she is born. Setting aside a few minutes each day for these sessions also helps everyone get used the idea of "special times" for learning after the baby is born.

**4)** Teaching your baby can be fun. It needs to be consistent, but it doesn't have to take a long time.

## Do I need to know if my baby is a boy or girl before I start the program?

No, you do not need to know your preborn baby's gender to participate in the Prenatal Classroom. However, there are many factors to consider when deciding whether or not you want to know your baby's gender before birth.

Sonograms, usually done in the fifth month of pregnancy, have become a regular part of many women's prenatal care, especially in countries where they are routinely available. During the procedure, it is possible to find out if you are going to give birth to a boy or a girl.

Some parents just can't bear the idea that they could know the gender of the baby before it's born or that someone else (the doctor, nurse, or midwife) knows the gender of the baby and they don't.

Before you agree to be told the gender of your baby, here are some issues to consider:

### Reasons for knowing the gender of your baby

**1)** If you know the gender of the baby, you can better prepare for gifts, clothes, nursery decor, and most important of all, which name you will choose for baby.

**2)** When you do your prenatal exercises, you can use the name you've chosen for baby.

**3)** You don't have to live with the uncertainty for more than five months about the gender of your baby.

**4)** If you have other children, knowing the gender of the baby will make him or her more real to them because it is not just a baby, it is a baby brother or a baby sister.

**5)** Your parents (and others) won't keep asking you if you know the gender or, if not, why you didn't find out.

### Reasons for not knowing the gender of your baby

**1)** Most gifts and clothes for newborns are interchangeable. If you get blue and want pink, it's easy to exchange. In some cases if you don't like a present, not knowing baby's gender gives you a good excuse to take it back to the store.

**2)** You may have preferred to have a girl and you are having a boy or vise versa. This may be uncomfortable for you and lead you to feel less connected with the baby.

**3)** Not knowing the baby's gender has a certain pleasurable climax to it when the baby is born and you find out what you got!

**4)** Your parents (or others) cannot continually ask about your expectations for the baby if they do not know the gender.

It is important for you to decide whether or not you want to know the baby's gender prior to birth. We believe it is best for you to make the decision based upon what you think is most appropriate. Stick to your decision and try not to let others' preconceptions sway you.

## How do I avoid gender stereotypes?

Whether or not we adults intend to, the way we relate to babies often reinforces gender stereotypes. We tend to encourage boys to move and explore and put them more frequently in simple, goal-seeking situations than we do girls.

Boys may hear, *"Let's see if you can reach the ball."* By contrast, girls are often placed in passive positions. The girl is told, *"Here is teddy bear. He wants to kiss you."*

Boys are given toy replicas of hammers, wheelbarrows, or cars, objects used to accomplish tasks. Girls are more frequently given nurturing-related items like dolls, toy dishes, or mirrors.

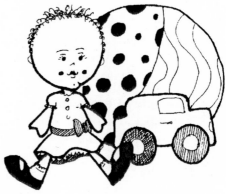

To avoid over-patterning your child's behavior after stereotypes, we recommend you frequently encourage your infant to explore his or her environment. Regardless of gender, provide the challenge of simple goals that are within your infant's capability.

## What are the basic principles of the Prenatal Classroom?

There are *eight basic principles* that form the foundation of the Prenatal Classroom philosophy and procedure. Understanding these principles will help you maximize your baby's potential to learn.

### The Cooperation Principle

Learning games and stimulation exercises help parents and other family members learn how to cooperate in working toward the baby's well-being before birth so they will know how to cooperate after your baby is born. This is true even if you already have had children. Prenatal Classroom exercises can improve cooperation between all participating family members.

### The Prenatal Bonding Principle

Prenatal Classroom exercises help prepare you for acceptance of your baby. Psychologists used to think that bonding didn't occur until after the baby was born. But by playing the learning games and doing the exercises, you can express affection and develop a bond of love before birth.

Dr. James W. Prescott has also reported that movement and touching stimulation helps your baby learn to give and receive affection.

### The Prenatal Stimulation Principle

A baby learns from stimulation. It is obvious to every new parent that tactile stimulation such as tickling, auditory stimulation such as the sound of mother's voice, and visual stimulation such as movements and colors become favorites for your baby throughout each day of his new, developing life. Prenatal Classroom exercises provide systematic stimulation for your baby's brain and neural development before birth. There is increasing scientific evidence that such activities help the baby's brain become more efficient and increase learning capacity after birth. The maximum growth in your baby's brain occurs before birth and up until he or she is about two years old.

### The Principle of Pre-Awareness

Prenatal Classroom exercises have the potential to teach your baby to recognize that his actions have an effect. In the Kicking Game, for example, when he kicks your abdomen in one place, your hand pushes back in the same place. The fact that this form of environmental stimulation can be taught before birth has tremendous potential in hastening your baby's learning about cause and effect after he is born.

### The Intelligence Principle

Albert Einstein is said to have responded to a question about his intelligence that "the secret of my great intelligence was that I have learned something new each day of my life." We believe intelligence develops from being interested in what happens and why it occurs. The Prenatal Classroom program includes exercises to interest your developing baby in sensations and sequences that can be perceived before birth. After birth, your baby may be more attentive and, therefore, has already begun developing his intelligence.

### The Principle of Developing Good Habits

You begin to develop good habits such as speaking clearly to your baby, expecting your baby to respond, and repeating exercises with good feelings when you do the Prenatal Classroom exercises. These good habits are then easy to continue once your baby is born.

### The Principle of Reassuring Siblings

By participating in the Prenatal Classroom exercises, your other children will feel important instead of neglected. They learn to expect that baby brother or sister will learn from them. This reassures your children that their place in the family is secure even when mother or father has less time for them.

### The Principle of Father's Essential Role During Pregnancy

Research has shown that good relationships between fathers and infants are strongly related to the child's development of social abilities. Since many of the Prenatal Classroom exercises can be done easily by fathers, and your baby will respond more to the deeper tones of the father's voice, we strongly recommend his participation.

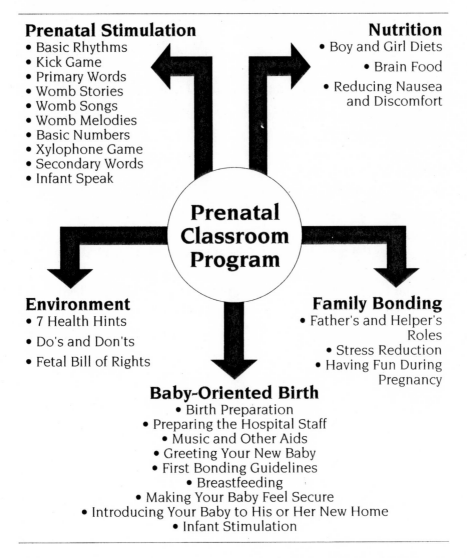

**Prenatal Stimulation**
- Basic Rhythms
- Kick Game
- Primary Words
- Womb Stories
- Womb Songs
- Womb Melodies
- Basic Numbers
- Xylophone Game
- Secondary Words
- Infant Speak

**Nutrition**
- Boy and Girl Diets
- Brain Food
- Reducing Nausea and Discomfort

**Prenatal Classroom Program**

**Environment**
- 7 Health Hints
- Do's and Don'ts
- Fetal Bill of Rights

**Family Bonding**
- Father's and Helper's Roles
- Stress Reduction
- Having Fun During Pregnancy

**Baby-Oriented Birth**
- Birth Preparation
- Preparing the Hospital Staff
- Music and Other Aids
- Greeting Your New Baby
- First Bonding Guidelines
- Breastfeeding
- Making Your Baby Feel Secure
- Introducing Your Baby to His or Her New Home
- Infant Stimulation

**A question to parents:**

## Why wait until your baby is born before trying to communicate with him or her?

In our experience, the time before birth is the best time to begin communication with your baby. It is a window of opportunity to reach out to your baby while there are fewer distractions in both of your lives. And it is during this period that your baby is developing faster than at any other stage of life. The positive habits you and your baby develop during the prenatal period of communication can last throughout childhood and beyond.

We do not maintain that if you use our program your baby will start talking, reading books, or dressing himself right after birth. However, your baby is capable of experiencing and learning before birth. If you start doing these early communication exercises before your baby is born and before you have the pressures of a newborn to care for:

1) It will be easier for you to become a playful teacher for your baby.

2) Other family members will feel involved with your baby before birth and will feel less threatened by your need to spend most time with the baby after birth.

3) Your baby will have the advantage of being reassured by familiar voices, sounds, and music after birth.

4) Your baby will have the potential to learn and form the connections about the meaning of what people say and do around him at an earlier age.

5) Your baby will be more confident because he or she will feel good about learning. A confident newborn feels good about learning to move, to listen, to talk, and to love.

# PART II
## A Healthy Pregnancy for a Healthy Baby

## Nutrition Guidelines Before and During Pregnancy

By deciding to participate in the Prenatal Classroom program, you are demonstrating an extraordinary commitment to the physical, mental, and emotional development of your preborn baby.

Nowhere is that commitment more vital than in the process of providing your preborn baby with the nutrition he or she needs to grow. You can start this process even before becoming pregnant by altering your diet and physical activity, if necessary, to provide baby with a healthy body in which to develop.

If possible, give your body a period of three to six months to prepare for pregnancy. During this time, you should eliminate all unnecessary medications like cold pills and aspirin and cut down on stimulants like caffeine. Stop smoking during this period and try to convince your mate to quit also because you "share air." If he smokes, you and the baby will still be receiving second-hand smoke.

Eliminate alcohol from your diet. Do not use marijuana or other drugs. Depending upon the kinds of drugs you may use, (either prescription or the unfortunate use of so-called recreational drugs) it could take several weeks for the chemical residues to leave your body.

Stop taking birth control pills several months before you plan to become pregnant, if at all possible. Birth control pills are known to increase chromosomal variations in cells and other abnormalities, which have the potential to adversely affect the fetus. You can use other forms of contraception until you and your partner are ready to conceive.

Be in the best shape you can be before becoming pregnant. This is the time to shed excess pounds, tone your body, and improve your cardiovascular system. Do *not* try to lose weight or increase your normal exercise regimen after you become pregnant.

Preparing for pregnancy also includes eating a nutritionally sound diet according to the guidelines that follow. It is an old cliche, but a sound one; during pregnancy you are not only eating for your health but for the baby's. In fact, the dietary recommendations in these pages are also designed to enhance your preborn baby's brain growth.

Following these guidelines will be easier when you learn which combinations of foods are best for you and your schedule of activities.

For example, working mothers may find cottage cheese combinations are easier to take to work for lunch than trying to find the right combination of foods at nearby restaurants.

You might want to consider consulting a registered dietician who could give you a number of specific menus that are right for you.

The dietary guidelines that follow are not meant to be used without modification or consultation with your doctor. This is especially true if you have specific food-related allergies or other dietary or metabolic considerations.

Recommendations to enhance baby's brain growth and development are not meant to contradict medical advice, should you have a specific nutritional requirement based upon a medical condition.

## Reducing Nausea

As with all guidelines in the program, use common sense in selecting foods and methods of preparation that best suit your preferences and how your body feels after you have eaten.

You would be surprised how many women complain of morning sickness, but never connect their queasy stomachs to the greasy fast food dinners they ate the night before. Maintain a list of what you eat and how you feel after you eat certain foods. If nausea becomes a significant problem during pregnancy, this list may be helpful to your doctor.

During your first few months of pregnancy, you will be more comfortable if you eat small meals frequently, rather than three large ones. This will decrease your tendency to feel nauseated.

## Transferring Taste

Give thought to what you eat during your pregnancy. Without realizing it, you may be creating a baby with a sweet tooth or a penchant for fried foods. One mother who participated in the Prenatal Classroom program reported she became a chronic doughnut eater during her first pregnancy. Doughnuts are high in simple sugars. After her little girl was born, the child's favorite food became doughnuts, and they still are to this day.

We believe that during the prenatal period, the flavor of foods can be transmitted to the baby. In his book, *Babies Remember Birth*, Dr. David Chamberlain describes how tastebuds start appearing on the tongue of the developing baby at the eighth week of gestation. By the thirteenth week, they have "reached adult form." All of the physical components needed for taste grow in within the following week.

Chamberlain goes on to say the fetus is capable of swallowing by the twelfth week.

"Putting this all together, scientists believe that your baby is having taste experiences for about 25 weeks before birth," Chamberlain writes.

As the food you eat is absorbed by your body, some flavor may cross directly into the blood stream and to the baby where he or she may experience it as a taste. If you eat a lot of one food during pregnancy, your baby may become quite familiar with the taste and actually prefer that food above others after birth.

So, odd as it might sound, don't be surprised if junior develops his Mommy's appetite for hot fudge sundaes or angel hair pasta with pesto sauce once you've started him on solids.

## Vitamin and Nutritional Supplements

Multi-vitamin supplements should be taken throughout pregnancy. While your doctor or health care professional should discuss your nutritional and vitamin requirements with you, we thought it helpful to include the following vitamin information.

### 1) Natural Vitamin E

Eat foods naturally rich in vitamin E. Natural vitamin E functions as an anti-oxidant and is meant to protect against "free radicals" which can produce chromosomal or tissue damage in your baby during the beginning stages of pregnancy.

| *Foods rich in vitamin E include:* | |
| --- | --- |
| wheat germ | egg yolks |
| whole grains | milk fat |
| green, leafy vegetables | butter |
| cottonseed, corn, and soybean oils | nuts |

### 2) Calcium

You will need to increase your calcium during pregnancy. Calcium is essential for the growth of your baby's bones and you will need to ingest more than is usual to avoid calcium depletion in your own body. Consult your physician for specific amounts you should be taking.

Physicians usually recommend 1,200 milligrams of calcium per day during pregnancy and while you are nursing. That amount of calcium cannot always be consumed in dairy foods such as milk, cheese, or ice cream.

Many women cannot rely upon dairy foods for calcium because

they are among the many people who when they were children lost the enzyme necessary to digest milk (lactose). If you are lactose intolerant and were to start drinking milk again during pregnancy, it might produce bloating, gas, headaches, and general discomfort. If you have a history of milk allergies, we suggest you reduce or eliminate the use of milk products during pregnancy, especially if you plan to breastfeed your baby. You may want to check with your local health food store regarding the different types of calcium that are available.

We recommend you supplement your diet with three to four calcium tablets each day. Taking calcium tablets prior to your pregnancy helps to build up a good supply of calcium for your body's needs.

There are several different types of calcium tablets to choose from. Calcium carbonate tablets contain 40 percent calcium. Calcium lactate tablets contain 13 percent calcium. Calcium Glutamate tablets contain 9 percent calcium.

One of the most convenient ways to take calcium is from chewable antacids such as TUMS. The product label contains the amount of calcium per tablet. Do not take antacids that contain aluminum salts, and as always, read the labels carefully. If you have any questions, ask your pharmacist to help you figure out the amounts.

---

*Good alternative sources of calcium include :*
    oyster shell calcium tablets
    turnip greens, 1/2 cup raw  246 mg.
    pink salmon, canned, 3 1/3 ounces  196 mg.
    white beans, 1/2 cup  144 mg.
    soybean curd (tofu), 1/2 cup  128 mg.
    almonds, shelled and dried, 1/3 cup  127 mg.
    fresh broccoli, steamed, 2/3 cup  88 mg.
    orange, 1 small  41 mg.
    egg, 1 large  29 mg.

* *mg. is the abbreviation for milligrams.*

---

### 3)  Iron Supplements

If you have a history of anemia or reduced iron stores in your blood, it is a good idea to supplement your diet with extra iron during the three months prior to the time you want to become pregnant. The extra iron will be stored in preparation for the rapid utilization during pregnancy when you will need more blood than usual, as well as meeting the rapidly increasing demands of your baby for iron. Consult your physician for proper dosage.

### 4) Mineral Supplements

Mineral supplements may be necessary if you have a diet high in processed foods and you consume few raw fruits and vegetables. When available or affordable, use fresh, organic vegetables and fruits in your diet before and during pregnancy.

### 5) Protein

We recommend you eat 85 to 100 grams (3 1/4 to 3 1/2 ounces) of protein each day from conception up to the 5th month of pregnancy. Beyond the fifth month, you can consume protein at your normal level.

The first 18 weeks is the time when brain cells increase from 125,000 neurons at 8 weeks to about 20 billion by the beginning of the 19th week. This is the highest number of brain cells that an individual will ever have during his or her lifetime.

A high-protein diet during the first 19 weeks of pregnancy has been shown to support the growth spurt of brain cells in the baby.

The protein can be from an animal or a vegetable source, as long as the protein source does not cause and/or increase nausea. For women who cannot tolerate red meats, we suggest trying turkey or chicken as the protein source. Try eating these with cranberry sauce. The cranberry, because of its high acidity, may help in digestion.

Gelatine capsules or plain, powdered gelatin may be mixed with fruit juice to ensure sufficient protein for women who will not or cannot consume meat, fish or fowl.

If you are using Prenatal Classroom's guidelines before becoming pregnant, start the high-protein diet about two months before you want to conceive. If you are using these guidelines after becoming pregnant, start consuming this amount of protein as soon as possible before the 19th week. You may stop consuming a high-protein diet after the 20th week of pregnancy.

### 6) Choline

Starting at about 18 weeks into pregnancy, we encourage you to follow a diet that includes a substantial amount of choline. Choline is a vitamin of the B complex found in both animal and plant products. It increases the ability of the baby's body to form rapidly growing neuron connections. Choline can be purchased in a pill form but is also found in several food products.

| Foods naturally high in choline include: | |
| --- | --- |
| egg yolks | peanuts |
| lean meats | beans |
| yeast | peas |
| soybeans | wheat germ |
| liver, brain, kidney, and heart meats | seaweed |

## 7) Water

Drink at least eight 8-ounce glasses of good water (check your source for contaminants, if possible) each day throughout pregnancy. This helps to carry away extra waste products and to replace water that is lost when you perspire. Perspiration increases during pregnancy.

The above guidelines are recommended for the health and well-being of you and your developing baby. It is not necessary for the rest of the family to eat in this fashion, but it is cheaper, easier, and more supportive if father eats the same foods as mother while at home.

## A Word About Vitamins and Nausea

Some women who experience vomiting from extreme morning sickness during the first four months of their pregnancy find that vitamins do not stay down and are not doing any good. If that is your situation and the vomiting persists, stop taking vitamins and notify your doctor immediately. Nausea is a normal symptom of pregnancy, but chronic vomiting could become a medical problem resulting in ripping of the stomach lining, severe nutritional and electrolyte imbalances, and even miscarriage. As soon as the vomiting stops, you should start taking the vitamins again upon consultation with your doctor. Chewable vitamins may help if you tend to gag when trying to swallow large capsules.

## Boy and Girl Diets

Research done in the early 1980s by Dr. Joseph Stolkowski at the Pierre and Marie Curie University in Paris, France, indicates women who increase their intake of certain nutrients before they become pregnant can influence the likelihood of conceiving a boy or a girl.

We have included diets based upon the results of Stolkowski's research for those of you who are more particular than others about the gender of your baby. Following these guidelines does not guarantee you will conceive the boy or girl you desire. But it doesn't hurt to try. As with the general nutrition guidelines, these boy and girl diets are not meant to be used without consultation with your doctor.

We recommend you begin the diet at least three months before you plan to conceive. The diet does not work after you conceive. While the male partner does *not* have to consume the diet, only the female, we again remind prospective parents that it is often easier and more supportive if father eats the same foods as mother while dining at home.

### Special diet to favor having a boy

Women who eat a diet high in sodium and potassium are more likely to have boys.

*Sodium is abundant in most foods, except for fruits. Foods naturally high in sodium include:*

    common table salt
    corned beef (or other cured meats)
    ham
    sausage
    seafood (especially tuna)
    pork
    luncheon meats
    soda crackers
    eggs

*Foods naturally high in potassium include:*

    beans, dried (cooked)
    lima beans
    white baked potatoes
    winter squash (baked)
    mushrooms (raw)
    beet greens
    radishes
    parsnips
    spinach
    peanut butter
    cantaloupe
    honeydew
    papaya
    apricots (fresh or canned)

**Special diet to favor having a girl**
Women who eat a diet high in calcium and magnesium are more likely to have girls.

---

*Foods naturally high in calcium include:*
   milk and milk products
   sardines
   clams
   oysters
   kale
   turnip and mustard greens
   broccoli

*Foods naturally high in magnesium include:*
   whole-grain cereals
   nuts
   meat
   milk
   green vegetables
   legumes

---

# Preventative Nutrition Before and During Pregnancy

1) **Salt foods to taste.** While we aren't recommending you cut back on salt, you may try tasting your food before you salt it to see if it needs as much salt as you normally use. Consult with your physician about your salt intake and any special medical problems which would require limiting how much you consume.

2) **Eliminate excessive caffeine** from your diet. Many products may contain caffeine (cola, other soft drinks, tea, coffee, chocolate, etc.). Read content labels carefully before purchasing and consuming any processed foods. *Note: Studies have shown that two cups of coffee per day had no adverse effect on pregnancy or miscarriage rates.*

3) **Avoid any foods you are allergic to** or which have given you discomfort in the past. If there are some foods which are more difficult for you to digest than others, you should avoid those foods during your pregnancy.

4) **Avoid excessive sweets and antacids.** The candies or antacids you take to calm an upset stomach may actually worsen morning sickness.

Instead, try eating acidic fruits such as lemons, limes, and cranberries, which will be better tolerated by your digestive system.

**5) Do not consume products that contain saccharin.** Warnings are printed on products that contain saccharin, a suspected cancer-causing agent. The effects of saccharin on your preborn are not fully known. Read labels carefully. Your Healthcare provider will be able to inform you about any new findings involving food adatives to avoid during pregnancy.

**6) Eliminate alcohol from your diet.** You should begin reducing the amount of alcohol you consume before you become pregnant and eliminate it altogether when you become pregnant. Drinking as few as one or two alcoholic drinks each day during pregnancy may result in miscarriage or a baby born with minor or major birth defects that are symptoms of fetal alcohol syndrome (FAS).

Babies born with FAS weigh less, are smaller, have small heads, and deformed facial features. Their IQ's are lower than those of their peers, and they may suffer from minimal brain malformations and dysfunctions, hyperactivity, joint and limb abnormalities, heart defects, newborn depression, and other behavioral disturbances.

Recent research also shows breastfeeding mothers who consume as few as one alcoholic drink a day can likely slow the development of their infants. If you currently use alcohol, you *must* discuss guidelines with your doctor.

**7) Stop smoking during your pregnancy.** The odds for a miscarriage occurring are greater if the mother or others living in the house with the mother smoke. The overwhelming evidence is that smoking causes lighter birthweight and increases the tendency of your child to have respiratory problems later in life by damaging the delicate breathing control centers of the developing baby. Sudden Infant Death Syndrome (SIDS) has been suggested  by some investigators to be related to possible effects of carbon monoxide from cigarettes on the respiratory centers of the developing fetus.

A study reported in the American Journal of Obstetrics in 1970 gives us some further understanding as to the remarkable communication and messenger service that goes on between a mother and her preborn child. Dr. Michael Lieberman showed that when a mother was asked to think about putting a cigarette to her lips (without actually doing it), the baby's heart rate went up and motion became more frequent and fitful. Increases in fetal heart rate are usually associated with some form of distress, so, perhaps, babies have also been trying to tell mothers to kick the habit.

**8) Eliminate any non-essential medications.** Medicines and drugs cross the blood brain barrier, which means that medicines that you take can affect the baby's brain and neural development. Ask your doctor before you take any medication while pregnant.

In the interest of a more natural life-style, many people now choose herbal remedies, teas, and other natural supplements for treating colds, allergies, and other problems. While this is an admirable intention, these substances are in reality medications, some of which may have harmful effects on the developing baby.

It is essential to understand that by growing up in a world filled with lots of easily available medicines, we have lost some of our sensitivity to how powerfully these medicines work in our bodies. Your developing baby is tiny compared to your body weight, and what affects a pregnant mother mildly may very well have a much greater effect on a preborn who quite simply hasn't got the mass to tolerate the powerful substances to which it may be exposed. You would not consider taking prescription drugs during pregnancy without first consulting your doctor. Do the same when you think about taking an herbal remedy or over-the-counter medicine.

**9) Do not take any recreational drugs while pregnant.** Stop taking any recreational drugs well before you plan to become pregnant. Do not take these drugs during pregnancy or while you are nursing. In addition to the harmful effect these chemicals have on the nursing baby, a drugged, less than fully aware mother trying to care for a newborn or toddler can be extremely hazardous to the well-being of the child.

During pregnancy, recreational drug use can cause a constriction of blood flow in the veins and arteries, which can in turn adversely affect your baby. Even casual usage of street drugs can profoundly affect fetal development, especially during the critical developmental periods early in pregnancy.

While often thought of as a "soft" drug, marijuana can also damage your baby's developing nervous system. Marijuana combines with neural receptor cells. While we really don't know what this will do to the baby's developing brain, we strongly suggest that this drug be avoided.

Most of us have not yet realized the awful time bomb that "crack babies" represent both to our society and to the future lives of these unfortunate children as they attempt to fit into society. Research has been able to determine complications associated with a pregnant woman's use of cocaine. These include high blood pressure, premature labor and delivery, and separation of the placenta from the uterine wall.

Those of us who believe it is important to protect fetal development from the adverse influences of medications and drugs in obvious cases such as babies who become addicted to crack during pregnancy will in the coming years need to take a hard look at our own use of convenience medicines and drugs that have become a part of our everyday lives.

# Environmental Do's and Don'ts For a Healthy Preborn

**1) Reduce the dust and pollutants in the air you breathe.** Because it is not practical for you to remove yourself from the source of pollutants (after all, you probably don't live on a mountain top), you need to clean the air around you. We recommend you use small negative ionizers (also called negative ion generators), which are very effective in removing pollutants from the air around you. They work by making dust particles (or pollen, cigarette smoke, chemicals found in smog from the freeway or exhaust from an industrial plant) clump together so they can be drawn to a spot where you don't have to breathe them. A small, powerful negative ionizer can be carried with you to be used both at home and at work.

Negative ionizers and H.E.P.A air filters are very helpful when you cannot avoid being around a cigarette smoker, such as a spouse or a co-worker. Even if you can't eliminate cigarette smoke or other air born pollutants, you can minimize your exposure to them as much as possible.

Many state and federal laws·govern smoking in public areas and workplaces. These have gone a long way in helping protect pregnant women and their developing babies.

**2) Avoid products containing potential toxins.** Reduce or eliminate the use of hair sprays, industrial cleaning fluids, oven cleaners, and other toxic products.

Many mothers toward the end of their pregnancy are driven by what has traditionally been called "the nesting instinct." They become obsessed with cleaning and preparing the nursery. This often includes painting the room or the baby furniture.

If you must paint, use water-based paint. However, we advise you paint before you become pregnant. Don't use petroleum-based paints or other solvents during pregnancy, if at all possible. These substances can be breathed and absorbed through the skin where they go directly into the blood stream, which, in turn, could harm your baby.

There have been many examples of people in confined spaces who have been overcome by fumes from oven cleaners, aerosols, and other solvents. Organic solvents used as anesthetics (at concentrations so low they could not be smelled) during surgery have been linked to increased rates of miscarriage in operating room nurses. As a result, hospitals across the country have installed air scrubbers to remove these vapors from operating rooms.

When cleaning the kitchen or bathroom, use only the mildest concentration of kitchen cleaners. Better yet, have your mate, a family member or friend do this kind of cleaning for you while you engage in other, non-chemical associated cleaning. Use caution and common sense when handling chemicals, cleaning or otherwise.

**3) Use pure water for drinking and cooking.** It is especially important to have pure water during your pregnancy because water which may be safe for adults may not be safe for a developing baby. Although most water supplies are safe, some city and public water supplies have been shown to be contaminated with harmful chemical waste. If you have your water analyzed and find it contaminated, you will need to find an alternative for drinking and cooking water.

Use purified water for drinking and cooking before and during your pregnancy, and as long as you are breastfeeding.

Bottled or spring water may be a good alternative if your public water supply is suspect. However, you need to be aware that different types of bottled water contain different levels of minerals. Some spring water is high in sodium (salt) and its use would not be encouraged in the later months of pregnancy. Others contain high levels of fluoride. Check which minerals are in the water you are considering.

Another alternative, and our recommendation, is reverse osmosis water filtration. With a small unit attached to your home water faucet, you can produce very pure water from your local tap water. Water filtration units using carbon filters are also useful, but not as effective as the reverse osmosis type.

**4) Avoid temperature extremes** in showers, baths, or hot tubs. Your developing baby cannot deal with temperature fluctuations and needs to be protected.

Natural temperature protection is provided for the baby by your body's regulation system which maintains your internal temperature even if the outside air temperature is cool or warm. If you enter a very warm bath or hot tub and you stay for a while, sweat will come to your brow. That is the sign that your body is working hard to keep your internal temperature down by releasing heat in the form of sweat. During pregnancy, you should get out of the tub before this happens.

Try not to expose the baby to temperature changes that may occur from sitting in a hot tub or bath or sitting in a sauna for too long.

Your body's temperature regulation system may also be stressed by swimming in excessively cold water or taking a walk on a particularly harsh winter's day. If your temperature regulation is overworked, then your baby, whose own system is not yet fully developed, will become even more stressed trying to balance the effects of the drastic change in his environment.

**5) Avoid loud noises** and sound levels above 100 decibels. Research has shown that noise above 100 decibels (the sound of a power lawn mower, chain saw, automobile, or noisy subway train) produces signs of distress in your baby. Loud rock concerts and stereo speakers turned to excessively high volumes are not recommended during pregnancy.

If you need to take noisy public transportation or work in a noisy environment, you can protect your baby by using padding such as a blanket to cover your abdomen. Obviously, you cannot eliminate noise from your environment, but you can and should reduce repetitive exposure to loud and disturbing noises.

Other cultures have long known about the detrimental effects of excessive noise on the developing baby. A 5,000 year-old Eastern writing called "Thaiko" that deals with the care and lifestyle of the pregnant woman advises: "The pregnant woman should avoid loud voiced arguments of men in the street and walk on the other side."

After you have used some of the exercises such as the Kick Game and the Primary Word List with your baby, you can use the same approach to prepare your baby before loud and frightening noises occur (when it is possible to do this). See examples in the Primary Word List using the words *loud* and *noise* for helping teach your baby to expect sudden loud sounds.

Hearing a loud sound every now and then won't hurt baby, as long as the sound doesn't exceed a decibel level that proves damaging to your eardrum. In fact, some medical centers use a device called an electronic larynx that produces a loud tone. Doctors use the larynx to startle the fetus and cause it to move in its mother's womb as a method of assessing fetal well-being.

While on the subject of fetal movement, you might find it interesting to know that the research of Eliahu Sadousky of Hadassah University in Jerusalem, Israel, suggests a preborn baby normally moves five times in 30 minutes. He goes on to say that if fewer than three movements occur in 30 minutes, you should listen for 1 1/2 hours to make sure a faster movement rate occurs. If in the last months of pregnancy fewer than three movements occur in eight hours, or fewer than ten movements occur in 12 hours, you should notify your doctor immediately.

You shouldn't have to startle your developing baby in order to feel him moving in your womb. Your baby will move normally without being startled. Following the simple Prenatal Classroom exercises will usually cause your baby to respond to presses on your abdomen, letting you know everything is just fine.

**6) Listen to the music that you enjoy.** While you are listening, your baby also will be responding to the music and will feel soothed and comforted. Dr. Susan Ludington-Hoe of the University of California at Los Angeles, and founder of the Infant Stimulation Education Association, believes this is true because the beat of the music is similar to that of your heartbeat. A selection of particularly calming music can be found in the appendix of this book.

The classical music of Mozart and Chopin seems to be especially soothing. We do not recommend loud rock 'n' roll or rap music which can irritate the baby. If you must listen to this kind of music, keep the volume down low and cover your abdomen with a blanket or pillow to insulate the baby from the noise.

**7) Try to avoid stressful encounters.** Although your baby can tolerate the occasional loud noise or stress of an argument, try to avoid too many situations like this. Your body reacts physically to stress by releasing brain chemicals which can reach and upset the baby. While it is virtually impossible to eliminate stress from your life, the stress reduction guidelines found later on in this book may help reduce a great deal of it, to both you and your developing baby's benefit.

**8) Try to reduce exposure to fluorescent lighting.** Some studies in animals have shown that excessive fluorescent lighting affects birth rates and contributes to birth deformities. Although no studies we know of have shown this in humans, it might be wise where possible to reduce the amount of your exposure to fluorescent lights, thus helping to reduce potential negative effects. We recommend that you use natural light-balanced bulbs which are available at most lighting stores. Also, try to spend time outside in natural light.

Other studies have shown that negative mood swings may be increased in those people who live in areas where there is little sun for long periods of time. In the far northeastern regions of the Soviet Union, where the people are deprived of sunlight for long periods, some suffer from Seasonal Affective Disorder (SAD), a depression that deepens through the winter months. There, schoolchildren "sunbathe" under ultraviolet light for a short period everyday to compensate for the lack of sun in their environment during mid-winter. The ultraviolet light also provides most of the vitamin D children's bodies need to fend off bone diseases and malformations.

Therefore, it is a good idea to spend time outdoors in natural light during your pregnancy. If you work in an office, try having your lunch outside a couple of times a week.

# Do's and Don'ts for Physical Activity

1) **Don't take up any new, strenuous sports during pregnancy.** As your pregnancy progresses, your body weight and center of balance change. Even experienced athletes can be fooled by small weight changes early in pregnancy. For example, skiing and horseback riding are two sports which require that you be able to change your balance rapidly, and in addition to the obvious physical peril inherent in both of these sports, should be avoided for this reason.

2) **Swimming is highly recommended.** Your body weight is supported by the water as you swim and, unless you are especially sensitive to chlorine, swimming will be a beneficial exercise during pregnancy. Because water is resistant to your body movements, it helps tone your muscles and improves your breathing.

3) **Low-impact aerobics consisting of easy, repetitive motions can also be beneficial** as long as the level of activity is not too strenuous. In practical terms, this means shorter workouts and more grounded movements, which reduces the possibility of falling, tripping or becoming overly tired or energy depleted. You can dance during pregnancy as long as you keep it simple and can maintain your balance.

Do not try crash programs to "get into shape" if you feel you are out of condition when you find out you are pregnant. Concentrate instead on slow and steady progress. Monitor how you change your movements as you gain weight, and you will learn to enjoy your exercise program and stick with it.

4) **Discontinue any activities which have been painful or which may**

**endanger the abdominal area.** For example, if you have had powerful, Swedish-type massages or if you took very hot baths after physical activity, you will need to modify those activities to make them more pleasant and less stressful during pregnancy. Trying to imagine what these and other activities are like for your baby inside the womb will help you change them appropriately.

Your baby can be injured by very violent starts or stops (as in an auto accident) without any blow or compression upon the womb. The internal force of the mass of the fetus and the placenta in motion at the time of the accident may be enough to inflict injury.

Some pregnant women express concern that wearing seatbelts may injure the baby. The exact opposite seems to be true. Wearing a seatbelt when traveling by car greatly reduces the potential for injury in an accident to both mother and preborn.

**5) Special exercise programs for pregnancy are a good idea.** These exercise regimens are tailored to your changing body and to preparing you for labor and delivery. Many hospitals and birthing centers have programs of this type, and we recommend your attending these classes if possible.

**6) Massage can be very helpful in releasing stress and toning muscles.** Massage can also be a good way for your husband or partner to keep and further develop the physical aspect of your relationship during a time when some women are insecure about their sexuality and sexual expression.

While you are using massage, refer to the Primary Word List in this book and add those words that fit what your baby may be feeling. Heavy pressure or deep tissue massage on the abdomen is not recommended during pregnancy. Some forms of yoga, like stretches, can also be beneficial.

**7) Nipple Stimulation.** Some pregnant mothers have been encouraged to rub their nipples with ointments or salves to make them tougher for breastfeeding. This is not a good idea.

Physicians, midwives, and nurses may have a woman rub her nipples in the "nipple stimulation test" when she is close to delivery or in the second stage of delivery to help with the delivery. This nipple stimulation is done to test fetal well-being because it causes pitocin (a pituitary hormone) to be released, which causes uterine contractions. If the nipples are over-stimulated for the purpose of toughening, contractions can be abnormally long and result in possible harm to the baby.

Rubbing of the nipples can also happen in sexual activity. If in late pregnancy any action such as rubbing your nipples or having them rubbed for sexual stimulation results in sensations that feel like contractions, it is very important that you stop this activity. You should discuss this with your doctor or other health professional.

## Traveling while Pregnant

If you travel during your pregnancy, the following simple suggestions will help you stay comfortable.

Don't take any long or difficult trips during the first three months of pregnancy. There is a higher than usual rate of miscarriage among women who travel during this time. Remember, if you travel to countries or places with different bacteria or viruses than you are used to, you and your preborn may become ill.

Drink lots of water when you fly. The artificial environments in airplanes tend to be very dry, and you can easily become dehydrated. Keep drinking water during the flight. If possible, bring your own pure water.

Avoid flying during the last six weeks of your pregnancy. The emotional excitement of preparing for and going on a trip may actually trigger labor in some women. Also, if the placenta is not functioning at proper levels of oxygenation and nutrition because of medical problems, baby may become starved for oxygen when the airplane cabin pressure is reduced.

## Protecting Your Back

One of the most common discomforts in the middle to late stages of pregnancy is lower back pain brought about by changes in your weight and posture.

Bending over to lift heavy objects without bending your knees is likely to strain the ligaments and discs where your back connects to your pelvis. Dragging heavy boxes while stooped over is another frequent cause of back injury. Back pain is of concern during pregnancy because the resultant discomfort may force you to take prescription pain medication repeatedly over the course of several days or weeks. The chronic stress produced by this recurrent and persistent pain, in addition to the chemical agents in the medication itself, may adversely affect your developing baby.

The best way to avoid back problems is to refrain from lifting anything heavy or at an awkward angle. Instead, ask your husband or someone else to lift objects for you. If you have small children who must be lifted and they are old enough to climb on a step stool or chair and stand up, help them to do that and then lift them up from the chair. This will keep you from having to bend over a great deal.

Whenever you are lifting something like a bag of groceries or a laundry basket full of clothes, face the load directly. Never try to lift something that's off to one side of your body. Keep your back straight, bend your knees to lower your body to a point where you can get a firm hold on the object and slowly lift it. Do not bend from the waist to lift.

# Reducing Stress and Minimizing Morning Sickness

### Stress Reduction

Planning for the birth of a baby should be one of the happiest times in the lives of both parents. However, it also tends to be one of the busiest. In addition to the demands of your regular schedule, you have to put together a nursery, see your doctor for regular medical check-ups, and attend birthing classes.

There is nothing wrong with being busy and having lots of things to do during your pregnancy. Whether this is your first baby or your fifth, you will need to make adjustments in your life-style. Whether for better or for worse, change is usually stressful because we humans are creatures of habit. But the last thing you want to be when you are pregnant is stressed out.

Your early pregnancy, before the baby is making demands on you as a parent, is a good time to learn how to let go of tension and prevent it from building up. The following two exercises provide a series of easy steps to help you release tension and reduce stress. That is why we recommend both the mother and father practice these steps together; you can share a quiet and peaceful moment away from the worries of your daily life.

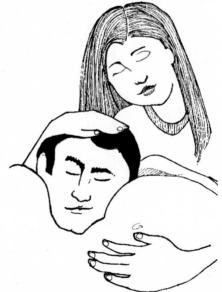

If you are having difficulty finding uninterrupted time, take the phone off the hook or shut yourself in the bathroom. If it is difficult to find a few minutes of free time now before your baby is born, you really need to learn these guidelines.

# Exercise A: Stress Release Breathing

INSTRUCTIONS

**Step 1:** *Loosen any tight clothing*, remove eye glasses or contact lenses, and do whatever else (remove shoes, for example) that is necessary for you to be able to rest and relax quietly for a few minutes.

**Step 2:** *Get into a comfortable position.* Try sitting, lying down, or lying on your side. As you progress through your pregnancy, you'll find that this position may change from time to time. In the later stages of pregnancy, you may find lying on your side more comfortable than other positions.

**Step 3:** *Identify any areas of tension or discomfort.* Pay attention to both your body and your state of mind. This will help you to identify an improved attitude or state of relaxation later.

**Step 4:** *Take 3 or 4 slow, deep breaths.* Make each breath a little longer than the last. Don't try to breathe in as much as possible. Instead, let the breaths seem to fill your abdomen first and then extend a little up into your chest. This is called "abdominal breathing." After the third or fourth breath, you should feel your body begin to settle down, relaxation is beginning.

**Step 5:** *Take 3 or 4 more slow, deep breaths, this time closing your eyes.* Notice that by paying attention to breathing out, the breathing in seems to happen all by itself. This results in a very natural, pleasing rhythm of relaxation breathing.

**Step 6:** *Identify the release and outflow of tension from your body and mind.* Although this effect will be more noticeable at some times than at others, it is important to practice the skill of releasing tension. Have you ever noticed your hands getting cold and clammy when you are under great stress? As the tension releases, you may start to feel your hands begin to warm. Hand warming is a good sign of tension release for most people. The circulation of the hands tends to mirror emotional condition.

**Step 7:** *In your mind, slowly repeat "Calm and peaceful, peaceful and warm."* Do this for about one minute. You can use any other words which represent for you the letting go of tension.

**Step 8:** *Picture a restful scene or imagine a good thought*, a memory of some place you like and find relaxing, or a fantasy image you find appealing. Concentrate on the good feelings for a few minutes.

**Step 9:** *Make contact with your developing baby by trying to visualize him or her.* Reassure your baby that you are doing your best to provide a safe and nurturing environment. Think good thoughts about making your pregnancy as good an experience as possible and having a wonderful and healthy baby. Some mothers like to visualize their babies at different stages of development, so we have provided an illustrated appendix for you to use beginning on page 43 that can help you visualize your baby during your sessions.

If there are unresolved emotional problems or things you need to change in your life, this is the time to talk about them with your baby, reassuring yourself and the baby that you are doing what you can to handle the present difficulty.

It is not important that you believe your baby can understand your concerns or thoughts. Just by spending this time practicing mental contact with your baby, you are forming a positive psychological bond. After your baby is born, you will be more likely to talk with him or her, which will make your baby even more responsive to you.

**Step 10:** *Prepare to open your eyes.* As you practice the first nine steps, you will become quite skilled at knowing when you have released tension and are ready to go back to your regular activities. As you open your eyes, stretch your arms down and breathe out through your mouth, making a sound of release. This alerts you to the resumption of your normal activities.

## Exercise B: *The Womb Journey*

INSTRUCTIONS

**Step 1:** *Pick a time* when you can be by yourself for at least 30 minutes.

**Step 2:** *Go into the bathroom* and draw a warm bath.

**Step 3:** *Take a radio,* preferably a battery-operated model, into the bathroom. Set it away from the bathtub or other places where it could get wet but within hearing distance. Never touch an electric appliance while any part of your body is touching water.

**Step 4:** *Turn the radio between stations to receive static.* Turn the volume down so that it is audible but not loud or disturbing. This static will produce what psychologists call "white noise," a relaxing, multi-frequency variable sound in the high range.

**Step 5:** *Turn the bathroom lights off,* or down low if you have a switch to dim the lights. When safely used, candles can have a wonderfully relaxing effect.

**Step 6:** *Remove your clothing and settle into the warm bath.* Get into a comfortable condition.

**Step 7:** *Close your eyes and let your mind go blank.* Try to imagine the sensations and the emotions of your baby floating in your womb. If any interesting thoughts about birth occur to your during this relaxation exercise, (or any other time, for that matter), you may want to jot them down afterwards. These thoughts can help you be more attuned to your infant during what we call the "baby-oriented birth," which will be discussed in a later chapter.

**Step 8:** *Remain in the warm bath* until you feel relaxed and refreshed.

While we hope difficulties in your life are minimal, we realize that some problems are unavoidable or unforeseeable. These are the times when stress reduction techniques can be lifesavers. One Prenatal Classroom mother put the techniques in the *Stress Release Breathing exer-*

*cise* to the test shortly after her baby was born. Dr. Van de Carr reports what happened:

*A young, first-time mother had used stress release methods to help with her delivery. When her baby was about three to four months old, she left the baby in the crib upstairs and went down to the basement to change a burned out light bulb. On the way down, she tripped and fell down the stairs and broke her ankle. As she lay in the darkness in intense pain, she could hear her baby crying upstairs. She suddenly remembered the stress release exercises and how she had used them to control pain during labor. She slowed her breathing, focused her attention and released tension, just as she had practiced a number of times before the birth. When she felt ready, she propped herself up on the stairs, crawled up the steps one at a time and then was able to continue crawling up to the bedroom where she reassured her baby and then telephoned for help. At that point, she realized that the pain no longer bothered her, and she waited calmly for the help to arrive.*

## Morning Sickness

Along with stretch marks and irritability, morning sickness is one side effect of pregnancy most women would rather skip.

The nausea and vomiting called morning sickness may occur at any time of day during your first trimester (three months) of pregnancy. Some fortunate women never experience morning sickness, but others find themselves "praying to the porcelain idol" everyday. (It also helps to keep your sense of humor about this typical symptom of pregnancy.)

We are not offering a cure for morning sickness. However, we do have a number of suggestions for minimizing the nausea you may be feeling. You will need to identify those particular practices which help you the most. We have developed this method based on the stress reduction guidelines just presented to help you.

To focus your mind on relieving the problems that may be contributing to your nausea, you need to put yourself in a calm and relaxed state. The instructions may appear identical to those for reducing stress, but your focus here is different from that exercise.

Pick a time to do this exercise when you are feeling as good as you can. Read the steps through to yourself several times until they seem familiar. Have your partner or a friend read them to you slowly so you will have time to carry out the thoughts or activity that accompanies each step. If it is inconvenient to have someone else do this for you, then use a tape recorder. Remember to space your steps so that you can go at your own speed.

# Exercise for Reducing Morning Sickness

**Step 1:** *Loosen any tight clothing*, remove eye glasses or contact lenses, and do whatever else (remove shoes, for example) that is necessary for you to be able to rest and relax quietly for a few minutes. If you have one of those convenient fingertip electronic thermometers, you can check your Fahrenheit temperature. (Fingertip temperature in the mid-80's° or below can be a sign of stress. 92-94° is considered to be a relaxed reading.) Or place your fingertip on your forehead. If your fingertip feels icy, cool or luke-warm to you, your hand temperature is less than 90° F. Test again after the exercise.

**Step 2:** *Get into a comfortable position.* Try sitting, lying down, or lying on your side. As you progress through your pregnancy, you'll find that this position may change from time to time.

**Step 3:** *Identify any areas of discomfort.* Pay attention to both your body and your state of mind. Don't fight discomfort; try to accept the sensations and let them pass through you. The less you fight against the sensations, the less tense you will be and the less discomfort you will feel.

**Step 4:** *Take 3 or 4 slow, deep breaths.* Make each breath a little longer than the last. Don't try to breathe in as much as possible. Instead, let the breaths seem to fill your abdomen first and then extend a little up into your chest. This is called "abdominal breathing." After the third or fourth breath, you should feel your body begin to settle down, relaxation is beginning.

Because of the discomfort and nausea you may feel, it is important to spend as much time as you need finding a way to let your breaths become slow and releasing. It may help you to imagine that with each breath out you are releasing some of the discomfort you feel. It is not necessary to go on to the next steps at this time. Practice as long as you like (usually 3 to 10 minutes) and as many times as you like.

Notice that by paying attention to breathing out, breathing in can seem to happen all by itself. This results in a very natural, pleasing rhythm of relaxation breathing. As your breath seems to come more from the abdomen, you will feel other parts of your body starting to release tension. It may seem as if your shoulders become heavier when tension is released from them. Your whole body may begin to feel heavy and warm.

**Step 5:** *Identify the release and outflow of tension from your body and mind.* Although this effect will be more noticeable at some times than at others, it is important to practice the skill of releasing tension. As the tension releases, you may start to feel your hands begin to warm. Hand warming is a good sign of tension release for most people.

**Step 6:** *Clear your mind to receive any messages your body may be trying to give to* *you*. Note any thoughts or ideas that may occur. Don't try to solve the problem, just wait to see if anything comes into your thoughts naturally. For example, you might realize that your clothing feels too tight, especially if you have not yet started wearing maternity clothes. Or, you may realize that you have to start changing your eating habits now that you are pregnant. Another message you may get from your body is to slow down and get more rest. Your body is going through a lot of changes in the first few months of pregnancy and even though they may not be noticeable on the outside, morning sickness may be a message to you to adjust your schedule and take it easy when possible.

**Step 7:** *Reassure yourself and your baby* that you will do the best you can to preserve your energy and enjoy those activities you still can do. It it important to remind yourself that good experiences and feelings occur during pregnancy and that there will be times when you are feeling better.

**Step 8:** *Picture a restful scene or imagine a good thought*, a memory of some place you like and find relaxing, a fantasy image you find appealing, or how you will feel in a little while when you no longer have morning sickness. Concentrate on the good feelings for a few minutes. Make them as real as possible for you right now.

**Step 9:** *Prepare to open your eyes.* As you practice the first nine steps, you will become quite skilled at knowing when you have released tension and you will feel much better. As you open your eyes, stretch your arms down and breathe out through your mouth, making an "*ahhhh*" sound of release. You are now ready to go back to your regular activities. Check your fingertip temperature again if you are using a temperature monitor. A good goal is about 92-94 ° which is very relaxed for most people, or if using your fingertip to your forehead, a feeling of warm or hot.

This technique has worked for many of our Prenatal Classroom mothers. At least one woman found the exercise not only made her feel more comfortable, it calmed down the whole family, as Dr. Lehrer reports:

*A mother in the beginning of the second trimester of pregnancy had a serious problem with morning sickness. As she learned to do these exercises, she reported that even when she went to her in-laws' house, which was quite chaotic with lots of children running around and making noise, she was able to sit quietly on the couch and practice her relaxation. This was quite remarkable to her because she was usually unable to stay in that living room for more than a few minutes before becoming sick. After doing the exercise on a few occasions, her nieces and nephew asked her to teach them how to do it. Things began to quiet down and become more peaceful for her during those family visits.*

When Dr. Lehrer read this example to his family as the book was being written, his oldest daughter Celene (age 8 at the time) drew the following picture about the woman practicing to help control her morning sickness.

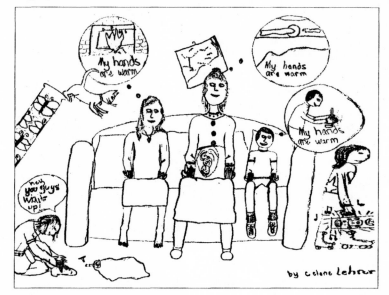

## A Fetal Bill of Rights

While it neither is nor was our intention to comment on the inflammatory issues concerning the legal status of the preborn in the United States or elsewhere, out of our interest in the issue of safety for the developing baby we drew up the first set of recommendations ever formulated to prevent excessive prenatal stimulation. We called these recommendations "The Fetal Bill of Rights."

We first presented these at the ninth International Congress of Pre- and Perinatal Psychology in Jerusalem in 1989. The Fetal Bill of Rights was meant to begin the process of addressing issues of fetal abuse.

Modern day society produces an environment that is increasingly unsafe for the developing baby. Excessive noise in urban areas, second-hand smoke, and low-level radiation from video display terminals are all potential and previously unknown hazards to which pregnant women are exposed at home and in the workplace. As a matter of fact, since our publication of the Fetal Bill of Rights there has been a number of research articles showing birth problems associated with long-term exposure to display terminals during pregnancy, and we are pleased to see some businesses adopting mandatory guidelines for pregnant women who use computer display screens at work.

Other environmental dangers include food and drinking water adulterated by chemical residues that at one time were thought to be safe but which are now being shown to have negative effects upon adults and their developing babies.

We bring these issues to your attention because we know anyone reading our book will do the best he or she can to prevent anything from harming their preborn children. This message needs to gain the widest attention possible if we are to prevent an unimaginable number of birth-related defects and avoidable maladies in the future.

# The Fetal Bill of Rights

Drafted by Prenatal University

Society's laws are meant to protect, not to harm, poison, or injure. Every day, in every country throughout the world, thousands and perhaps millions of preborn children are needlessly denied their natural opportunity for normal development.

Prenatal University calls upon the concerned people, parents, educators, and lawmakers of every nation to recognize once and for all the opportunities available to the preborn child.

We hold these truths to be self evident. That every preborn child has:

**1)** The right when the fetus becomes a sentient being to have an unobstructed prenatal development.

**2)** The right to have adequate nutritional support to develop a healthy mind and body.

**3)** The right to be protected from exposure to poisons and toxins that retard neural and physical development.

**4)** The right to a healthy womb environment free of physical trauma or harmful levels of noise, light, or other excessive stimulation.

**5)** The right to be accepted as an individual, alive and aware before birth.

If you believe as we do in the absolute necessity of establishing the above opportunities for the preborn child, the coming generations will respect and thank you for your courage and protection.

# 7 Health Hints For a Good Pregnancy

1) Follow the general pregnancy diet described in this chapter until your 19th week of pregnancy.

2) Try to rid your environment at home and at work of possible contaminants that may harm your developing baby.

3) Don't smoke during pregnancy. Remember that if you or your husband smoke, your chances of miscarriage are greater.

4) Don't drink alcoholic beverages during pregnancy. Check over-the-counter medication (such as cough syrup) which may contain alcohol.

5) If you experience morning sickness or queasiness, eat several small snacks throughout the day rather than three large meals.

6) Unless your physician advises against it because of a specific health risk, continue to exercise (walk, stretch, ride a stationary bicycle, or do specialized low-impact aerobics) throughout your pregnancy.

7) Practice your abdominal breathing and visualization exercises.

# Prenatal Classroom Visualization Images of Your Developing Baby

Many parents tell us that they like to imagine or visualize their pre-born's development while doing the Prenatal Classroom exercises. By doing the visualization exercises and imagining what your baby looks like, you can begin sending positive thoughts of love and affection while holding these images in your mind.

The illustrations and time frames given below are approximations of how your preborn looks at the given time.

## 6 Weeks After Conception

At this time, you will test positive for pregnancy. At this stage your baby is just beginning to develop the spinal areas and brain. The tiny heart begins to beat. Even though your preborn doesn't look much like a baby yet, all the necessary developmental forces are at work to help the preborn grow.

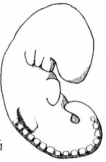

*Baby's size - less than 1 inch*

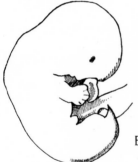

## 7 Weeks After Conception

Little nubs or bumps start to appear, which will eventually develop into hands and feet. Baby's head and neck begin to take shape.

*Baby's size - 1 inch*

## 8 to 9 Weeks After Conception

Baby makes his or her first small movements, but you can't feel them yet. Your preborn has eyes (but no eyelids), and ears are beginning to form.

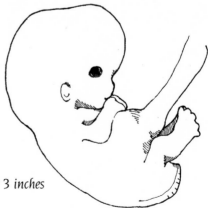

*Baby's size - 2 or 3 inches*

## 12 Weeks After Conception

Now your preborn is starting to look more like a baby. The head is very large in proportion to the body and taste buds are mature. Olfactory nerve (part of the brain related to sense of smell) is fully developed. Facial expressions begin to develop.

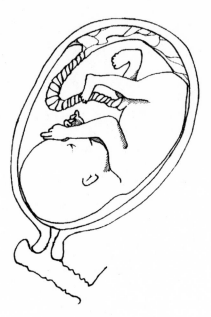

*Baby's size - 3 or 4 inches*

## 14 Weeks After Conception

Your baby can now perform internal physical functions like swallowing. Baby reacts to internal fluctuations in temperature and can differentiate between sweet and bitter tastes. He or she has tiny fingernails and toenails. Eyes are becoming sensitive to light. You are probably beginning to see the slight bulge of your pregnancy.

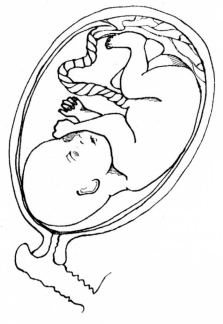

*Baby's size - about 5 inches*

## 18 Weeks After Conception

Your baby can now close his or her eyes, and is starting to grow eyebrows, eyelashes, and hair on the head. Now or within 3 to 4 weeks, you will begin to feel your baby move. Baby's brain development accelerates and convolutions begin to appear. Mother may be able to feel baby's hiccups.

*Baby's size - 8 inches*

## 22 Weeks After Conception

Your baby begins to have definite sleep and wakeful periods that you can perceive. In addition to your heartbeat and other internal biological sounds, your baby can now hear sounds from outside of the womb. Baby is now sensitive to touch.

*Baby's size - 11 inches*

## 26 Weeks After Conception

Baby is now covered with a thick protective coating called "vernix." Baby's kicks become more pronounced and frequent. Baby's weight has doubled during the last 4 weeks. REM (rapid eye movement) can be detected, baby may be "dreaming." Baby becomes more responsive to sounds.

*Baby's size - 13 inches*

## 30 Weeks After Conception

Your baby's lungs are maturing in preparation for his or her first breath of air. Baby may be sucking his or her thumb by now. Baby is now big (and heavy) enough that mother is walking by leaning back with legs slightly apart to keep her balance. Baby can now move in rhythm and may show preferences for particular musical selections.

*Baby's size - 15 inches*

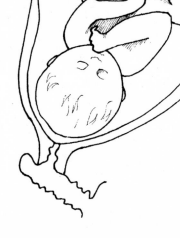

## 34 Weeks After Conception

By this time baby has assumed the head down position and no longer has room to turn or somersault about. Kicking is pronounced, and you may be able to observe movements of hands and feet. Baby can respond differently to mother's, father's, and other family member's voices.

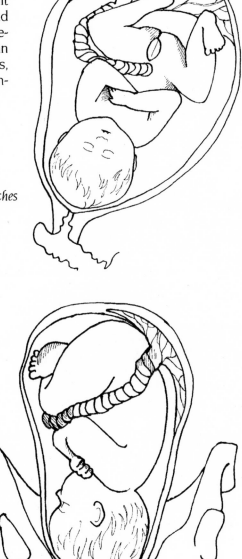

*Baby's size - 17 inches*

## 38 Weeks After Conception

Your baby is considered "full-term" now. The head drops down toward your pelvis in preparation for birth. *Both you and baby are ready for birth!*

# PART III
## *Prenatal Classroom Curriculum*

# First Communication Exercises With Your Baby

The first part of the Prenatal Classroom program is geared towards getting your baby to recognize that a repeated stimulus (something that you do on a consistent basis) can have both pattern and meaning.

You will begin at the end of the first trimester by introducing your baby to a series of repetitive drum rhythms. Throughout these exercises, baby discovers the existence of rhythms other than mother's heartbeat. The exercise is also the first step in teaching your baby about the world outside the womb.

By the fifth month of pregnancy, your developing baby should be ready to learn *verbal* (sound) and *tactile* (touch) communication. You will begin the lesson by teaching baby to respond to your voice and with gentle pushes on mother's abdomen in the Kick Game.

The fifth month of pregnancy is a natural time to begin a touch relationship with your developing baby. This time is very special because it is when mothers begin to feel the baby as both a physical and an emotional reality. Baby's rapidly increasing size makes mom suddenly look bigger, and baby's independent motions in the womb can be felt and even seen through mom's abdomen. For some new parents, this is the time when the baby becomes "real."

*I am reminded of a mother who prior to her first pregnancy had a Siamese cat named 'Miss Kitty.' Miss Kitty was treated as a baby and was even fed from a baby bottle. The cat was hugged, held, wrapped in blankets, and taken on vacations. Miss Kitty was very much this woman's baby even during the early months of her pregnancy. One day in the fifth month of her pregnancy, she noticed Miss Kitty playing on the floor with a moth. Kitty played with the moth for a while, and then ate the moth. The mother-to-be suddenly looked up in horror and exclaimed in a loud and surprised voice, 'Miss Kitty is an animal!' and asked her husband to 'put the cat out'. Her husband said that, at that point, she was rubbing her abdomen as she spoke. Thus we see a natural emotional transfer of affection from the surrogate baby (Miss Kitty) to the fetus that often occurs in the fifth month of pregnancy.*

(Dr. Van de Carr)

### Being Consistent

Learning how to be constant and consistent when stimulating your baby is more important than the variety of stimuli you are providing.

This principle will be repeated throughout the exercises.

For example, when introducing your baby to the Primary and Secondary Word Lists in this chapter, avoid using two different words for the same object, action or person. As adults we frequently do this, calling the same piece of clothing a "coat" at one time and a "jacket" at another time. But using different names for the same thing may confuse your preborn baby and prevent him from learning.

Along these lines, it is best if you decide what you want baby to call you after birth, and stick to that name throughout the exercises. We suggest you use "Ma Ma" and "Da Da" because these words will be easier for your baby to say than "Mommy" and "Daddy" when he or she starts talking.

It is important that everyone identify themselves in their own voices. A common mistake, for example, is mother telling the baby, "That's your Da Da talking," or "Da Da is going to talk now." Only Daddy himself should use the word "Da Da." Your baby is still learning to match the voice with the sound of the word. If you have children that also want to talk to the preborn, make sure each one identifies only himself or herself in a natural voice to the baby.

*Carefully read through the instructions before you begin an exercise.* While most of the exercises require little more than your hands and voice, some of them require certain materials like a xylophone or a small drum. We will provide guidelines that explain what to do, when to do it, and what materials you might like to use. Some exercises have a • **tip** section that can help explain different aspects of methods in an exercise. Some even have a **Variations** section because we feel that certain exercises have an element of flexibility in which parents and baby can find what suits them best.

## How to Talk to Your Baby

With the exception of the drum rhythm and musical exercises, all of the Prenatal Classroom lessons require you to talk to your baby through the womb. That means you must learn to talk so that baby can hear you.

Although your baby is capable of hearing when you are about 18 weeks pregnant, sounds from outside the womb are filtered through mother's abdomen and through the liquid sack of the placenta in which baby is growing. You have to direct and amplify your voice to reach those tiny ears.

Because some mothers speak softly, we recommend they use a megaphone, a rolled up piece of paper, or a hollow tube to help project their voices toward their abdomen. A good, loud voice can also do the trick, but you don't need to shout or yell.

*I thought that my baby could never hear my regular voice, so I got the idea to roll up a newspaper as a megaphone to make it so my baby could hear me. Dr. Van de Carr congratulated me and said I didn't need a lot of expensive equipment to be able to talk with my baby before it was born.*

(Comment from one of Dr. Van de Carr's Prenatal University participants)

If you are not using a megaphone or similar device, you need to speak at about two times your normal conversational volume. This is about the same as talking loudly enough to be heard by someone on the other side of a room, 15 to 20 feet away (approximately 80 decibels).

Mothers, if you speak a bit more loudly than is usual, project your voice towards your baby, and can feel your words vibrating through your body, then your baby will hear and feel the words too.

Bring your head down toward your abdomen and project your voice towards your baby. Don't try to bend or force your neck down in any way that does not feel comfortable for you. That is why we recommend using a tube or a megaphone. We want you to enjoy the process rather than feel like you are trying to stretch your body more than is right for you.

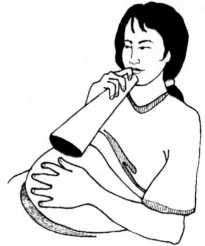

The technique is different when it comes time for Dad or another helper to do the talking. Your helper can place his cheek on your abdomen close to where the baby's head is located and talk directly to the baby. A helper who is speaking to the baby with his cheek on your abdomen can speak at a normal volume as if he were talking to someone standing a short distance away. Your helper should speak conversationally in a natural and reassuring voice, pausing occasionally as if he or she expected the baby to answer.

Another effective method for communicating with your baby is for mother to lie in a bathtub of warm water with her chest and neck beneath the water and her chin just above the surface. The walls of the bathroom and the water surrounding the abdomen and throat tend to magnify mother's voice, making it easier for baby to hear. In this position, you will not need a megaphone or other device to project your voice.

Of course, if you are in this position, a helper should not put his head underwater. Amusing as it might be, it doesn't really accomplish much. Instead, he should moisten his cheek with water (for better sound conduction) and place that side of his face on your abdomen just over where the baby's head and ear are located. See page 62 for finding baby's position.

## Closing with Music

If possible, finish each session with some music, singing, or humming. Play the music on a small, portable tape recorder or music box. Sing or hum a special song you like to your baby.

Whichever method you choose, finish each communication session with two minutes of the same piece of music when it is convenient to do so. This helps create definite boundaries for the rest of baby's day. Your baby will learn that a period of stimulation is followed by music and then a period of rest. Using this music while your baby is quieting down after an active period will help your baby learn to associate this music with relaxation and comfort.

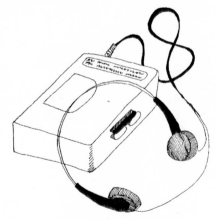

Because transition times are similar to times of drowsiness in the newborn infant, this will also help establish a regular sleep cycle for your baby after birth. In our experience, this same music played to babies intermittently during labor and delivery is very beneficial. It calms the babies and reduces the trauma of the birth experience.

If you are singing or humming, you will not need to use the megaphone since the baby will be able to feel and hear the vibrations from your singing. Volume is not so important here. If a helper is singing, he should put his mouth close to your abdomen so that the baby will pick up the vibrations from the song. If you use a tape recorder or a music box, be sure that the volume is not too loud. Music that you find relaxing and soothing will probably soothe your baby as well. Pick tunes that you like, or make up your own. Musical selections that we recommend are listed in Appendix B at the end of this book.

## When to Begin Practicing

Guidelines for when to begin are given along with each individual game and stimulation exercise, and an overview of suggested times and sequences for all of the games and exercises is provided at the end of this chapter. If you enjoy a particular activity or the baby is more responsive to it, you can do it more often. If baby doesn't respond to a certain activity, do it less or try again in a week or so.

If you are starting the Prenatal Classroom program after the 20th week of pregnancy, we recommend you begin with the Kick Game for ten days, with two sessions each day. Give baby the experience of kicking paired with the word *"kick"* four times each day, ideally two kicks for each session. You can then continue with the Kick Game while beginning other exercises.

# Heartbeats and Drum Rhythms

From the moment of conception, your baby feels its mother's heartbeat. This is the first awareness that all of us have.

Even before the auditory organs develop, the baby grows with the feeling of the ever-present, pulsing heartbeat. This basic pulse is an essential part of our being. We begin our lives sensing the pulse, and after we are born the memories remain deep in our consciousness.

This beat may act as a biological metronome as the brain and body begin to grow and organize. Some preliminary research by Dr. Brent Logan, Director of the International Society for Prenatal Learning and Bonding, suggests that varying the frequency of the applied heartbeat sounds may help stimulate neuron connections in the preborn baby's brain, resulting in better intellectual performance.

Your baby can also be introduced to rhythms outside mother's body through Prenatal Classroom exercises. Of course, the baby will not be physically capable of hearing these rhythms during the first months of pregnancy, but he or she will be able to feel the vibrations.

Later in your pregnancy, the baby will be able to hear the rhythms as well as feel them. Our findings and those of other researchers indicate infants in the womb can, in fact, hear noises from outside the mother's body starting at the 18th week of pregnancy.

Dr. Van de Carr discovered firsthand that babies in the womb can and do react to the rhythms that enter their environment at a far more sophisticated level of awareness than was previously believed possible:

*I had an interesting observation during the pregnancy of one my patients several years ago that also shows how preborn children respond to music and rhythms.*

*I usually keep a small stereo tape player in my examination room. During an ultra-sound examination, I played a tape of Beethoven's Sixth Symphony. I was watching the baby's rhythmic chest movements, which are a type of pre-breathing that may occur naturally in the womb during the third trimester of pregnancy. I suddenly became aware that the breathing movements were exactly timed to the beat of the music. I pointed this out to the mother who also observed the movements. She had played Beethoven's music at home for the baby and one of her favorites was the Sixth Symphony.*

*I then stopped the music, and the baby's chest motion stopped! I waited.*

*No movement!*

*I started the music again, and the movements started but not in time with the music. One breath, a second breath, a skip and then suddenly the chest movements were again in exact time with the music. I repeated this several times for the mother and myself to observe.*

(Comment from Dr. Van de Carr)

One Prenatal Classroom mother reported that after her baby son was born he responded in an unusually favorable way to an annoying sound he had remembered hearing before birth:

*Two mothers, who are friends, took their one-month old infants to visit the husband of one of the women at the automobile body repair shop where he worked. This was the first time the wife had visited her husband at work since the baby was born. As they entered the shop, a large and very loud air compressor suddenly turned on. One baby was quite startled and began screaming and crying (a very normal response). But the baby son of the mechanic looked around slowly at the machine and smiled. The wife of the auto mechanic had visited the shop many times during her pregnancy. Her baby, while still in the womb, had become accustomed to the sound of the air compressor. His smile may have been a response of recognition as he discovered the compressor was the source of this familiar sound.*

(Dr. Van de Carr)

These outside sounds – father's voice, music, the rumble of a car engine – are muffled as the sound waves pass through mother's womb. Your baby is literally underwater, hearing the sounds made by the objects and creatures in the unknown world above. Our research shows deep, baritone voices can penetrate the barrier of the womb more successfully than higher pitched voices. By the same token, your baby will hear the deep plunk of a bass or the thump of a drum more clearly than the whistle of a piccolo.

For this reason, we recommend you introduce baby to his or her first external rhythms by playing them on a small drum placed on mother's abdomen. You can begin this exercise by the end of the first trimester. However, at any point from conception on, you can begin to use rhythms in a consistent way to interact with your baby.

This is done by mother or mother's helper beating the small drum in a slow, consistent pattern. The goal of this exercise is to teach the developing baby a primitive understanding of patterns. This use of rhythm is just a variation of the patterns produced by mother's heartbeat that the baby has been – and will be – feeling throughout the pregnancy.

Many musicologists believe the rhythms and time signature of most music has its origin in the human heart rate of about 60 beats per minute. This is why babies are most often soothed by classical music of Chopin, Mozart, and Vivaldi who consistently used tempos that are reminiscent of the human heartbeat.

We also find this same effect in paintings where the soothing images of mother and child show the infant held on the left side where he can hear his mother's heartbeat.

Prenatally stimulating your baby using music may also influence his or her own musical talent. Our colleague, Dr. Donald Shelter, a jazz musician and a professor of the Eastman School of Music at the University of Rochester in New York, has been researching the effects of playing symphonic musical selections to babies before birth. A large percent of his subjects (children aged 2 years and younger) could use one finger to play notes on a piano rather than bang away at the keyboard as most young children do. These children were also quite good at picking out simple melody patterns.

Similar research has now been started in Japan with similar initial results. We have also heard comments from family members that suggest another kind of connection:

*I always danced to music with you before you were born. Maybe that's why you always had such a good sense of rhythm.*

(A 70-year old grandmother talking with her 35-year old daughter in Dr. Lehrer's office after he told her about the Prenatal Classroom program)

Most so-called primitive cultures use rhythms and dance as a natural part of tribal life. Pregnant women do repetitive dances to ritualized music throughout their pregnancy. Their preborn babies become familiar with the sounds of the rhythms and the feelings of movement associated with these rhythms prior to birth. After birth, the babies continue to hear the rhythms which are already familiar to them.

Be it tribal song, Top-40, Beethoven's Sixth, or television theme songs, developing babies are highly discriminating listeners and can pick out minor variations in tone and melody.

A study conducted in 1989 in Belfast, Ireland, showed that 12 women who spent more than six hours each day watching soap operas delivered babies who quieted down when they heard the soap opera themes. This is an example of prenatal conditioning that goes on all too frequently in our modern society. Is this the prenatal conditioning we want for our babies?

In contrast to contemporary culture, Joseph Chilton Pierce in his book, *The Magical Child* (1977), describes how non-urban Ugandan mothers massage, caress, and sing to their infants in the first two days after birth. These babies were "awake a surprising amount of time, alert, watchful, happy, calm, and they virtually never cried."

In speaking with a Ugandan physician who worked in rural areas, Dr. Van de Carr discovered that the mothers sang along with ritualistic swaying and movement during pregnancy. These motions, coupled with sound, are similar to exercises we will have you do in a later section.

Swaying, singing, and ritualized movements and rhythms are also a part of other African cultures. Nigeria, for example, has specific dances, movements, and songs to perform throughout pregnancy, according to Babatunde (Baba) Olatunji, a master Nigerian percussionist and director of the international Nigerian Dance and Drumming group.

In Western culture, we have lost touch with many of the ritualized sounds, rhythms, and dances with which even our grandparents were familiar. Instead, we are far more likely to have our preborn babies exposed primarily to the sounds of television themes, ringing telephones, and the movements of elevators, automobiles, streetcars, and buses.

When the pregnant women is at work she is also likely to be inactive for long periods at a desk or computer terminal. Too much inactivity can subject babies to a kind of sensory deprivation.

For these reasons, we strongly encourage families to sing songs, dance, and play music together during and after pregnancy. The singing and musical accompaniment that goes on during religious services is often repetitive and can be soothing or stimulating to your baby as well as helping to develop heightened rhythm and musical ability.

55

## Simple Drum Rhythm Exercise

**Goal:** To present a consistent vibration (and sound) the baby can feel.

**Materials needed:** A small drum. The Native Americans of the Southwest make little cottonwood drums that are great for this exercise, but drums that can be found in children's toy stores work just as well. The drum does not need to be played loudly, but it is best if it has two heads, so that hitting it on one side creates a vibration on the other side.

**How to do the exercise:** Place the drum over the abdomen so that one side touches your belly. Hit the drum with a stick or mallet so that it creates a sound and so that you can feel the vibration on your abdomen as well.

**When to begin:** You can begin the use of simple rhythms or music any time after conception. However, we recommend these vibration rhythms be started after the 18th week of pregnancy when the baby has developed the ability to hear.

**How often the exercise should be done:** Simple drum beats should be done twice each day. We recommend 30 minutes to two and one half hours after eating as the best time to do the rhythms. That's because your baby, having received nutrients from food you digested, will be more awake and alert than at other times. Preborn babies are frequently alert after dinner from 8 to 11 p.m.

If your meal includes foods with a high sugar content, you may expect your baby to become active sooner than when your meal consists of starches, which are more slowly digested. When your baby doesn't have enough sugar, he or she tends to be quiet, sleepy, and relatively non-reactive in the womb. Even the baby's heart may tend to show fewer variable rhythms. In hospital tests to check the baby's well-being, we frequently give the mother a dose of sugar in orange juice to see if the baby's heartbeat becomes more variable and the baby moves more in the womb.

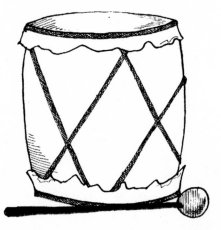

## Simple Drum Rhythm Exercise

**1)** *Start with a simple two-beat rhythm.*

**Step 1:** Hit the drum, pause one half of a second and then quickly hit the drum again.

**Step 2:** Pause 3 seconds, then repeat the two drum beats.

**Step 3:** Repeat the whole sequence for about 1 minute.

*Use this simple two-beat pattern for one week.*

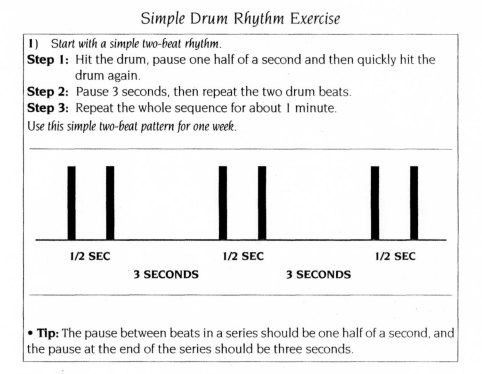

| 1/2 SEC | 1/2 SEC | 1/2 SEC |
| 3 SECONDS | 3 SECONDS | |

• **Tip:** The pause between beats in a series should be one half of a second, and the pause at the end of the series should be three seconds.

## Changing Rhythms Over Time A

**2)** *Start with a simple three-beat rhythm.*

**Step 1:** Hit the drum. Pause one half of a second and then quickly hit the drum again. Pause one half of a second and then quickly hit the drum again.

**Step 2:** Pause 3 seconds, then repeat the three drum beats.

*Use this simple three-beat pattern for one week.*

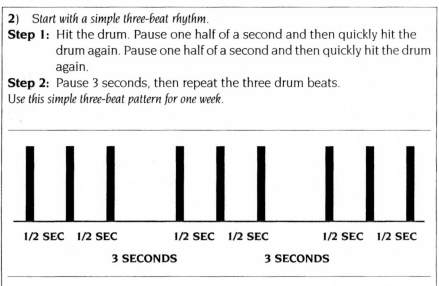

| 1/2 SEC | 1/2 SEC | 1/2 SEC | 1/2 SEC | 1/2 SEC | 1/2 SEC |
| 3 SECONDS | | 3 SECONDS | | | |

**3)** *Alternating three beats and two beats – 3 second pause*

**Step 1:** Hit the drum. Pause one half of a second and then quickly hit the drum again. Pause one half of a second and then quickly hit the drum again.

**Step 2:** Pause three seconds.

**Step 3:** Hit the drum. Pause one half of a second and then quickly hit the drum again.

**Step 4:** Pause three seconds.

**Step 5:** Repeat the whole sequence for about 1 minute.

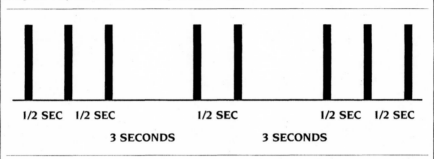

| 1/2 SEC | 1/2 SEC | | 1/2 SEC | | 1/2 SEC | 1/2 SEC |
|---------|---------|---|---------|---|---------|---------|
| | 3 SECONDS | | | 3 SECONDS | | |

• **Tip:** Vary other patterns or repeat any of the above patterns throughout the pregnancy. Whatever pattern you use, repeat it consistently for about a week to give your baby the idea of a definite pattern. Do not try to create complex patterns. You may find that your baby "likes" some patterns more than others.

Music and rhythms can stimulate different areas of the brain related to language and mathematical development. As you practice these rhythms for your baby, you yourself may also be developing some new skills and appreciation of musical patterns and rhythms that you can share with your baby after birth.

# The Kick Game

### Baby's First Interactive Learning Game

Around the beginning of the fifth month, you'll start to feel little kicks or movements in your lower abdomen. Kicking at this time is entirely normal. This is your baby's way of beginning to explore and to learn something about his or her world. Because the baby is floating inside the womb, connected by the umbilical cord and occasionally touching the sides of the uterus, the only way for him or her to make contact with the outside world is through some kind of kicking action.

Kicking also helps strengthen your preborn's legs. It's nature's built-in exercise program. Many parents who have used our program have noticed their babies' legs seem particularly strong when compared to other children's.

In the Kick Game, your baby will learn the basics of responding to others. It's a simple game – your baby kicks and you gently pat or press the spot on mother's abdomen where she kicks. Once the baby has become accustomed to your pats in response to her kicks, you can start saying the word "*kick*" when you pat.

If you consistently pat mother's abdomen in response to her kicks, she may begin to kick more at certain times and in certain places. After three or four weeks of playing this game, you might try moving your pat over a few inches, and see if she kicks where you have moved your pat!

*When I was about six months pregnant, we noticed that if my husband patted, our baby would kick where he patted. By the eighth month, we had taught the baby to follow my husband's pats in a circle. It was amazing.*

(Comment from another excited mother who had verified in her own home the baby's learning process)

Since 1982, we have had more than ten reports of seven to eight month old prenatal babies who would kick in a circle. In all cases, both mother and father really enjoyed the exercise. Beyond the parents' amusement, this example shows that the baby is no longer simply kicking in a random fashion, but has learned to move his point of contact with the mother's womb to match the pattern of exterior pressure applied by the father.

We welcome parents' little improvisations to further explore their developing baby's capabilities. The concepts of Prenatal Classroom exercises are simple enough that some parents have even been able to perform them based upon cursory explanations in newspaper and magazine articles. One such couple living in Taiwan read about the Kick Game in an edition of the "China Post," an English-language daily newspaper. They tried the exercise and were able to start tactile-verbal communication with their baby midway through the pregnancy. The baby's father sent Dr. Van de Carr a letter:

*Since January, my wife and I have been experimenting with the Kick Game with very encouraging results. I can certainly say we are getting a big KICK out of the exercise! So far we are in the sixth month and our baby is responding almost too well. A few nights back I asked, 'Who is the greatest father?' and received a quick kick in the ear.*

(Todd Waldman, Feb. 20, 1986)

## The Kick Game

**Goal:** The purpose of the Kick Game is to teach your baby that his actions will elicit a response and are a way of communicating.

As you progress to more advanced variations of the game, the baby will learn that actions can be repeated and that they are connected to certain words. In the Kick Game your baby learns to respond to two kinds of outside stimuli – tactile (*touch*) and auditory (*sound*).

An additional goal of the game is to teach parents to be aware of baby's activity and almost instinctively respond to it.

**Materials needed:** A megaphone, a rolled up piece of paper or hollow tube, or just your louder than usual voice projected down toward your abdomen. If another family member is saying "*kick*," he or she can be quite close to your abdomen and can direct the voice right to the baby.

**When to begin:** You can begin the Kick Game when you are about five months or 20 weeks along (or any time between the fifth and seventh month if you begin Prenatal Classroom instruction later in your pregnancy). After about a month or when you notice that your baby consistently responds to your words and actions in the Kick Game, you can start doing the more advanced versions. Continue to play the Kick Game for at least one month and stop any time after the seventh month.

Even if you do incorporate the Kick Game into your stimulation sessions after the seventh month, you may continue to play it occasionally, even during the later months of pregnancy. It's fun.

**How often the exercise should be done:** Usually the best time for the Kick Game is about 30 minutes to two and a half hours after you have eaten a meal. Play the game for about two minutes, two to three times each day.

You do not need to respond to the baby's motions or kicks every time they occur. It is more important to pick times when you can give your attention to responding.

**• Tip:** We all have times when we are distracted and just go through the motions of doing something without really paying attention to what we are doing. If something else is on your mind at the time when the baby is moving and you want to play the Kick Game, take a minute or two to clear your thoughts before you begin. Then play the Kick Game and afterwards go back to what you were doing. This way you will get used to the idea of giving your full attention to your baby when it is needed. Then you can return to other activities.

# The Kick Game

**Step 1:** When the baby starts to make kicking motions:

    **a)** gently pat or press your abdomen with one hand where the baby is kicking. Do this part of the Kick Game whenever you like. Get used to responding to the baby's movements.

    **b)** after several days, begin adding the words *"kick, kick"* at the same time you are patting back.

*For Mothers:* Direct your voice, rolled paper tube, or the megaphone towards your abdomen.

*For Helpers:* Put your cheek directly on the abdomen with your mouth close to the baby's head when you say *"kick, kick."* Mothers, tell your helper when and where the baby is kicking. He will then press or pat your abdomen and say, *"kick, kick"* when the baby kicks you. Do this two or three times as the baby kicks.

**Step 2:** When the baby starts to kick back where you have been pressing or patting your abdomen, you can press back again and talk to the baby. This may happen quite quickly or take some weeks – try not to be impatient. Sometimes the baby refuses to play at all. As long as your doctor assures you that the preborn is healthy and developing normally, this is no, repeat, no cause for alarm. Remember, every baby is unique and responds differently.

    Say "Hi, *this is Ma Ma. Kick. That's a good baby. Kick here again."*

Wait for another kick and respond to it in similar fashion. Repeat this once or twice.

## Variation 1

    As with the other steps, a helper also can talk directly to the baby. If the helper is Dad, he would say, "Hi, *this is Daddy. Kick here. That's a good baby. Kick here again."*

    When you say *"kick here"* you are patting where your baby has just kicked. Some parents like to have fun and say "Kick Ma Ma. *That's a good baby. Kick Ma Ma here."* This may seem like a strange thing to say, but we are only trying to teach baby to associate some specific sounds and actions. In this case, it's the kicking movement associated with the word *"kick"* and with a location *"here"* or "Ma Ma."

• **Tip:** The baby is starting to get the idea that the physical sensations related to kicking (your pressing of mother's abdomen in response) are associated with certain sounds (your saying "Hi, *Kick Ma Ma,"* etc.). Although you are not trying to teach the baby words at this time, it is very important that you be consistent in what you say and that you talk to the baby in the same way you would to someone who is listening to what you say and who you expect to respond.

**Step 3:** Finish the Kick Game sessions by playing soft music with a regular beat, such as Chopin, for the baby if it is convenient to do so.

## Advanced version of the Kick Game

> If and when baby responds to your pats and words with kicks, you can make the Kick Game more interesting.
>
> INSTRUCTIONS
>
> **Step 1:** Wait until the baby is kicking and responding to your pats and presses. Move your hand several inches to a new area of mother's abdomen you believe will be easy for the baby to move towards and press and pat in this new spot.
>
> • **Tip:** It is not unusual for the baby not to respond at first. Go back to pressing where the baby is kicking and try moving in a different direction.
>
> **Step 2:** When the baby does follow your presses, say, *"Good! Kick here again."*
>
> **Step 3:** After awhile, you can make a very advanced game by moving your presses in a circle or other pattern for the baby to follow.

# Second Phase – Advanced Learning Games

The beginning of the seventh month (28 weeks) of pregnancy is the best time to start the second phase of the Prenatal Classroom program. We call this the second phase of the program because you already have made some prenatal contact with your baby by using the rhythm exercises and the Kick Game. Now you can begin to "teach" your preborn.

The second phase consists of additional exercises based on the same communication principle as the Kick Game, but now you begin introducing simple words and actions. For example, you will say *"pat, pat, pat"* while patting mother's abdomen, or *"rub, rub, rub"* as you rub mother's abdomen in a circular motion.

Remember, in these sessions it is important to practice talking to your baby and expecting a response. This is a two-way communication, and you need to be aware of your baby's responses as well as your own.

We suggest two sessions per day. Try to plan one session in the morning which you can do alone, and one in the evening with Dad or another family member participating. Five to ten minutes per communication session should be enough. A communication session consists of as many of the advanced learning games, with the exception of Infant Speak, as you wish to include.

If you especially enjoy a particular activity or your baby is very responsive to it, you can do it more often. If your baby does not respond to a particular activity, you can do it less often, or stop and reintroduce it about a week later.

Select a sequence for the various games and exercises and maintain it from session to session. There is some evidence to suggest that your baby will remember the pattern of what you do. Changing that pattern may be confusing. In other words, if you start with the Primary Word List and then go on to the Xylophone Game, you should keep that order during subsequent sessions.

Use common sense in doing only as many activities as fit comfortably into your schedule. When you enjoy what you're doing, your baby will sense that this is worth knowing and doing.

All of the following games and exercises can be started at about seven months or 28 weeks of pregnancy. Specific guidelines can be found with each.

# Finding Baby's Position

**Goal:** To do some of the advanced learning games, you will need to find the position of your baby in mother's womb.

Finding the position of the baby should be done only after 28 weeks. His or her position cannot be easily or reliably determined before that time. In general, the baby's back will lie opposite the side where the mother usually gets kicked.

If the mother is unusually heavy, it may be difficult to determine the location of the baby even after 28 weeks and up until delivery without special diagnostic techniques.

**Materials needed:** None

**How often the exercise should be done:** When the directions for the learning games that follow tell you to pat, rub, or tap a certain part of the baby's body, first find that part of the baby and then continue.

**Things to keep in mind:**

**1)** When you are undergoing a prenatal physical examination, pay attention to the techniques and amount of pressure used by your doctor, midwife or nurse. When the time comes for you to check the baby's position yourself, remember how it was done during your examination.

• **Tip:** During one of your routine office visits, ask your doctor to show you where the baby's head and back are located. If for some special reason you are having an ultra-sound examination, you will be able to actually see the position of the baby in your womb.

**2)** When feeling for the different parts of the body – head, back, and bottom – do not push so hard that you hurt or even cause discomfort to yourself. If the pressure is uncomfortable for you, it may also be uncomfortable for your baby. Because you want learning to be pleasant for the baby, it is important to avoid any unpleasant sensations. If you press in and out gently and quickly on your abdomen, you will be able to feel the baby's body parts moving back and forth against your fingers. Using this method you won't have to push as hard to feel the baby.

**3)** If you determine baby's position at the beginning of a stimulation session, you do not need to recheck it during the session unless you feel the baby shift position.

**4)** As a general rule, baby's back will be opposite where you are most frequently kicked by the baby. If the baby is kicking you in the same general area (and the back is in the same area) as you determined during the previous session, the baby has probably not moved.

**5)** If you are at all unsure about the position of your baby during the later stages of your pregnancy, please ask your doctor for instruction at your next office visit.

• **Tip:** At this time in your pregnancy, the baby tends to move from its position less often, and you should not have to check baby's position all the time.

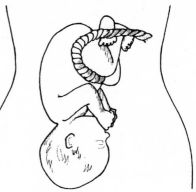

In this view, you see the baby in its normal upside-down position. Approximately 95 percent of all babies will lie in this position. If you find that your baby feels as if it might be in a different position, head up in a breech position for example, ask your doctor about it.

## Breech Position

If, while doing these exercises, you notice that on several occasions the firm ball-like part (baby's head) is at the top of your womb and the soft, rounded part (baby's bottom) is down low, you should call it to your doctor's attention. This is called a "breech position." In only about 4 percent of pregnancies are the baby's head in the upper part of the abdomen and the feet toward the lower part.

If your baby is in the breech position, do the rubbing and patting exercises on the lower part of your abdomen. The stroke exercise would be done from the top of your abdomen down. This strokes the preborn baby's back from top to bottom.

## Two Babies or More

If you know that you are going to have two babies or more then it may be difficult to know where each baby is located.

Because there is less room in the uterus–we recommend checking more frequently with your Healthcare provider about using any of the Prenatal Stimulation exercises especially during the last month of your pregnancy. Most parents of twins have been able to use these methods with success.

### Finding Baby's Position

INSTRUCTIONS

**Step 1: The baby's bottom.** To find the baby's bottom, use one hand to feel the top of the womb at just about the point of your naval. The baby's bottom will feel soft and rounded and seem to be an extension of the legs. When you feel the baby's bottom, it will seem to move less than other parts of the baby. The baby's bottom is at the top of the womb as is shown in the figure below.

• **Tip:** The bottom should be opposite and slightly below the point where you most often feel baby kicking.

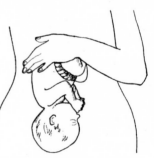

In this view, you are feeling the top of the womb for the baby's bottom. The bottom will feel soft and round and seem to be continuous with the back.

**Step 2: The baby's back.** The easiest part to find is the baby's back. Hold your hands with the fingers pointing downward. With one hand, feel for a long, smooth area of firmness, probably off to one side of your abdomen. With your other hand, try to find the baby's arms, which feel like small, well-defined lumps.

If the baby's back is on the right side of your abdomen, use your right hand to locate the back and your left hand to feel the small, lumpy parts. If the baby's back is on the left side, use your left hand. The back should be on the side opposite to where you feel the baby's short, quick kicking motions. Don't be confused by the baby's long, slow stretching motions, which you may feel on both sides.

The following figure shows you how the baby is lying inside the womb and how to position your hands to find his or her back.

• **Tip:** A general guideline is that the baby's back will be opposite to where you usually get kicked.

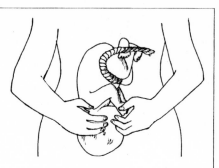

In this view, one hand (in this case the left hand) feels for the small, lumpy parts that are the baby's arms while the other hand feels for a firm, smooth area that is the baby's back.

**Step 3: The baby's head.** There are two methods to help you locate the baby's head.

**A)** Place both hands over the lower abdomen just above your pubic hair. Move them back and forth, feeling for a firm, rounded form bumping your fingertips as you move hands.

**B)** In the second step, you will use one hand. Press gently just above your pubic hair. If you feel a firm, round ball, this is the baby's head. Gently push in and out, feeling the fullness of the baby's head beneath the palm of your hand. Let your fingers slide more deeply around the head.

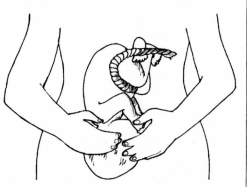

View (A) You are feeling for a round ball lying in the abdomen just above the pubic hair. You are moving your hands gently back and forth and feeling the mass of the baby's head as it bumps your fingers.

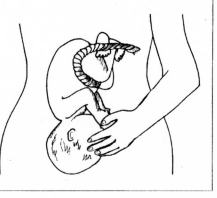

View (B) This is a one-handed check for the position of the baby's head. The palm of your hand should feel the firm head beneath while the fingers slide around the margins of the head.

# Educating Your Preborn

## Congratulations!
## You and Your Baby Are Now Learning Together

You start each session with the following two steps. After you have finished these, you will be ready to begin the Prenatal Classroom Second Phase learning games.

*Entering the Prenatal Classroom*

INSTRUCTIONS

**Step 1:** The best way to physically arrange yourself for the session is to lie on your back, turned slightly so that your weight is on the left side. This position tends to increase circulation of blood to the womb, which will benefit the baby during the communication time. Of course, you also may sit, stand, or arrange yourself in other positions, depending upon what is possible for you at the time and what other activities you are involved with.

## Variation

Another very effective position is for you to lie in a full bathtub of warm water with your chest and neck beneath the water and your chin just above the surface. As we mentioned earlier, when you are in the tub you should not need a megaphone or other device to project your voice.

**Step 2:** As you start to talk to the baby, identify yourself in your own voice. Keep it simple, say something like, "Hi, *this is* Ma Ma."

## Variation

If Dad, or another family member is going to start the session he would say:

"Hi, *this is* Da Da."

"Hi, *this is* brother, Bill."

"Hi, *this is* sister, Mary."

• **Tip:** As with the Kick Game, mother needs to speak about three times louder than usual. Helpers should place their mouths near the baby's head and speak in a natural voice at twice the normal volume. See the section **How to Talk to Your Baby,** to review methods for talking to your baby. Remember, part of the exercise is your learning about getting used to and setting aside special times for talking with your baby.

Now you are ready to begin the first advanced learning game, The Primary Word List.

# Primary Word List

## Your Baby's First Vocabulary Lessons

Each word on the Primary Word List describes a sensation that your baby is capable of feeling inside your womb. The words are divided into groups according to the kinds of sensations they describe. Some of the words have a tactile or touch quality that your baby can feel, such as *kick* as is used in the Kick Game. Other words are associated with sound, motion, or visual stimulation.

The Eskimos have over twenty words to describe different types of snow, while North Americans possess in their lingual repertoire hundreds of phrases to describe automobiles that would bewilder a Kahlahari Bushman, for whom *car* would suffice. Cultures make and use words that describe things that are important to them. Prior to the Prenatal Classroom program, the only word that English-speaking mothers commonly used to describe actions that babies made in the womb was *kick*. As you will see, there is room for improvement in this particular area of our language.

In the Prenatal Classroom we want you to become sensitive to the number of experiences that your baby has in the womb and give names to those experiences. When you do this you are not only practicing the words with your baby, you are also increasing your awareness of the baby's expanding consciousness. Once you start to think this way, you may discover other words that represent your baby's experiences and motions.

Although you may select some additional primary words of your own, it is very important that each word be associated with its own stimulus. For example, don't say *"pat"* when you use a rubbing motion or *"rub"* when you use a patting motion. Changing the stimulus and subsequent events will confuse the baby and will make learning unnecessarily difficult.

The first five words on the list, those associated with touch and vibration, are the most important. The baby becomes familiar with your touch, your voice, and the very motion of your body as he or she floats inside your womb. In a paper entitled "Phylogenetic and Ontogenetic Aspects of Human Affectational Development," Dr. J.W. Prescott writes that these sensory experiences actually stimulate the growth of brain cells that are responsible for the ability to give and receive affection. Without development of the brain's "affection center," a person would be biologically incapable of such a basic human emotion as love.

## The Prenatal Classroom 26 Primary Words

All the words in the first group convey a *sensation*. Because they are tactile, your baby can feel all of these actions when you do them.

A pat feels different from a rub or a shake or a squeeze. When you first start to pat or rub your baby's back, he begins to learn the difference between a pat and a rub because they *feel* different to him. After a while he starts to recognize the sound of the word *pat* as meaning the sensation that he feels when you pat him. In the same way, your baby will begin to learn the sounds of all of the first 6 touch-related words on the Primary Word List:

1) **Pat**
2) **Rub**
3) **Squeeze**
4) **Shake**
5) **Stroke**
6) **Tap**

Words in the second group convey *motions*. When you practice these your baby is learning about movements. They are:

7) **Up**
8) **Down**
9) **Sway**
10) **Rock**

The third group of words conveys *sounds*. When you play music, run a vacuum cleaner, or attend a fireworks show, your baby is listening. Your baby is learning to recognize different sounds. As you continue stimulating your baby, he will learn to recognize the sound of the word *music* with the experience of music. These auditory words are:

11) **Music**
12) **Loud**
13) **Noise**

The fourth group of words conveys the *sounds and sensations associated with mother's and baby's biological functions*. Baby cannot only hear your cough, he or she can feel the vibration in your chest. When you hiccup, baby can feel a quick contraction of your abdomen. He or she can experience more complex biological interactions when you cry or laugh. These "complex sensation" words are:

14) **Cough**
15) **Sneeze**

16) **Hiccup**

17) **Cry**

18) **Laugh**

Words in the fifth group convey a *visual* sensation. Even though many people don't know it, it has been recently discovered that your baby can see before he is born. We use the words *light* and *dark* because your baby can easily recognize the difference between these two visual experiences.

19) **Light**

20) **Dark**

Words in the sixth group convey a *thermal* sensation that your baby can begin to recognize late in pregnancy. The two words you will be using are:

21) **Cold**

22) **Hot**

Words in the seventh group involve *movements that baby makes*, which you can feel. We have already introduced the first of these, *kick*, in the Kick Game. These words are only practiced when you feel the baby do them. Anytime you feel your baby kick, hiccup, or push (seems to stretch out in your womb), you can say the word that you feel your baby doing. It is not necessary for you to respond all of the time, just when you feel like it.

23) **Kick**

24) **Push**

25) **Roll**

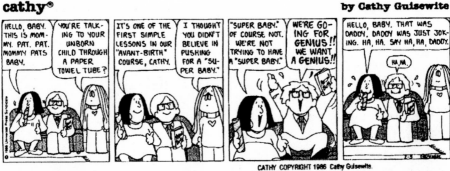

cathy®                                                by Cathy Guisewite

CATHY COPYRIGHT 1986 Cathy Guisewite.

Reprinted with permission of Universal Press Syndicate. All rights reserved

*Part III: Prenatal Classroom Curriculum* 70

## "Not" – the 26th Primary Word

You can teach your baby about opposites by using the word *"not"* in front of some of the other primary words.

For example, once you have practiced the word, *"shake"* and its accompanying sensation with your preborn, you can say *"not shake"* right after you stop shaking your abdomen. Or, you can pair *"not"* with the word *"noise."* Say *"noise"* and turn on your vacuum cleaner. Then switch off the vacuum cleaner and say, *"not noise."*

• **Tip:** If you find that you are doing the exercise in a mechanical way, just repeating the words, then more than likely it's not the right time to play the game. Perhaps something else is on your mind. Please remember, our experience in showing these exercises to thousands of parents has taught us that they work best when they are enjoyable for the person who is doing them. This also means that you don't have to do all the exercises. We have included in the Prenatal Classroom a complete set of exercises that covers all of the activities that many different mothers and fathers have used. Just like in any school, you, the teacher(s), have a choice about which parts of our learning guide you want to use and what modifications you want to make to those exercises. Naturally, don't use any exercise that makes you feel uncomfortable.

## Primary Word List

**Goal:** To teach your baby to associate specific sensations with specific words. This is done by using words that describe actions or sensations that the baby can experience inside your womb.

**Materials needed:** A megaphone, hollow tube, or your own projected voice (nice and loud), a portable cassette tape player or radio, a halogen flashlight, and a hand-held massage unit (optional).

**When to begin:** Any time after the seventh month or 28th week of pregnancy. You will continue the Primary Word List in modified forms through birth and early infancy.

**How often the exercise should be done:** When you first use the Primary Word List, we recommend you repeat the whole list two or three times during each session. If you can't do all the words, (for example, if you don't have your flashlight for *light* and *dark*), just do as many as you conveniently can. After you have become more practiced, you can run through the list, once per session. Going through the list should not take as long once you have become more experienced. At this point, (at about 4 weeks of practice), you may start trying some of the variations that will be described later. Working mothers report that they often practice some of the Primary Words while sitting at their desks or during short breaks.

## The Primary Word List
### Level 1: Words associated with touch

The first words you can teach your baby all have specific touches or movements that your baby can feel at the same time he hears the word. As you repeat the words and the movements during a period of four to six weeks, the baby will begin to make associations between your touch and the words. This will better prepare him to understand words after birth.

We are not saying your baby will understand the Primary Words after he is born. However, repeated exposure to the words while in the womb can move up the age at which your baby will be able to recognize and understand them in early infancy. In our research and in the research that other investigators have now reported following our work, prenatally-stimulated babies recognize words and demonstrate verbal skills much sooner than those youngsters who were not prenatally-stimulated. They also pay attention to what their parents say to them because they expect the words to make sense.

---

**1) PAT**

Locate the baby's back or bottom as described in **Finding the Position of Your Baby**. The back will usually be found in the upper part of your abdomen. If the baby's head is in the upper part of the abdomen and the feet lower down, (breech position), pat the lower part of your abdomen. Holding your fingers together, pat your abdomen using the palm of your hand.

*Pat* is a firm yet gentle contact with side of your abdomen where the baby's back or bottom is located. You should be able to hear the sound of the pat, but the impact should not be uncomfortable for you. About one second after you pat the baby, say the word *"pat"* in a clear, firm voice. Repeat this several times.

• **Tip:** When first starting, you pat or rub the part of baby that you can feel most easily in the upper part of the abdomen. This is usually the wide part which is the baby's back or buttocks. As you learn the activity over several weeks and as the baby continues to grow, it should become easier for you to determine the back and buttocks. In about 4% of pregnancies the baby's head is in the upper part and the feet are toward the bottom of the abdomen. Your health care provider will know if this is the case after the 28th week of pregnancy. This is called a breech position. In this case, do the rubbing and patting lower on the abdomen.

*Variation*

As you advance in using the primary words and when you become familiar with the location of the baby's body, you can begin teaching baby about different body parts. Example: *"Ma Ma pat back," "Ma Ma pat head."* etc.

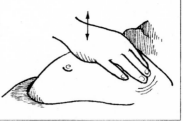

---

## 2) RUB

Locate the baby's back or bottom. Using the fingers and palm of your open hand, rub the side of your abdomen where the baby's back or bottom is. Rub in a circular motion using slight pressure. As you rub the baby, say the word *"rub"* in a clear, firm voice.

*With my first child, my husband would rub my stomach every night at 10 o'clock and rub the baby's back. The baby would move under-neath his hand and calm down, which would then let me sleep. After the baby was born, we noticed that if she was upset or cried, she would calm right down or go to sleep if he rubbed her back.*

(Comment from a Prenatal Classroom mother about her baby's sensory memory)

## 3) SQUEEZE

Place your hands on each side of your abdomen, feeling for the baby's body and head. Use only your fingertips when locating your baby's position. Placing your hands on either side of the baby, apply pressure with both hands, gently but firmly squeezing the baby. Be sure to use the heel of your hands when doing this. Use even pressure that builds slightly and then slowly lets up. This should be less pressure than your physician or midwife uses during clinical exams. This sensation will be somewhat similar to what the baby will feel during a contraction in labor.

As you squeeze your abdomen, say *"squeeze"* in a clear voice. Say it slowly, making it take about two to three times as long as usual (*"squeeeeeeeze"*). Drop your voice a little at the end of the word. By dropping your voice, you are giving a non-verbal (tonal) message that the pressure from the squeeze is also stopping. This will be similar to the sigh of relief that will be occurring during labor.

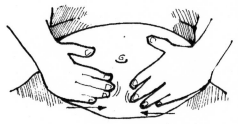

• **Tip:** Never squeeze hard. It should be comfortable for you.

73

### 4) SHAKE

Locate the baby's back and bottom. Place both hands on either side of your abdomen where the baby's back and bottom are. Move your hands up and down while saying "*Shake, shake, shake.*" Let your abdomen fall back into place after you have lifted it.

Shaking should always be done with both hands. The movement is a series of up and down motions that last for 2 to 4 seconds. Let your abdomen fall back into place after you have lifted it. At first, repeat the series several times. To be consistent, the word "*shake*" can be repeated each time you lift your abdomen. Say, "*shake, shake, shake, shake, shake,*" then pause and repeat, "*shake, shake, shake, shake, shake.*"

• **Tip:** Grasp your abdomen firmly but do not push hard. It should be comfortable for you.

## Variation 1

After 4 weeks of practice, you can shake fast or slow, and you can say "*shake fast*" or "*shake slow.*"

## Variation 2

Also after 4 weeks of practice, you can use a hand-held massager to teach aspects of the word "*shake.*" Place the massager against the side of your abdomen on the firm area where the baby's back is.

Turn it on and  say "*shake fast.*"
Turn it off and say "*off*" or "*not shake fast.*"

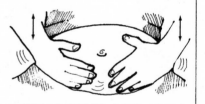

When using a massager in this way do not leave it on your abdomen for more than 5 to 10 seconds at a time. Use only a battery powered massage unit and do not take it into the bathtub with you.

### 5) STROKE

Place your fingers over the area where the baby's back is located, but near the bottom of the abdomen. Move your hand upward while maintaining pressure against the baby's back until you have reached the upper part of your abdomen, which will also be the baby's bottom if he or she is lying in the head-down position.

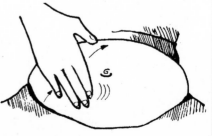

As you stroke your abdomen this way, say "*stroke.*" Repeat several times, stroking your abdomen each time you repeat the word "*stroke.*" You can also elongate the  word,  "*strooooooooke.*" Accompany the word with a slow, strong movement.

### 6) TAP

Locate the baby's head. Hold your index finger up in a slightly bent position, then bring it down against your abdomen in a rapid motion. If you want to know how this will feel to your baby, ask someone to use this tapping motion on the top of your head while you cover your ears. However, baby has lots more additional padding between the head and the tapping finger than you do.

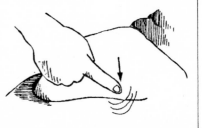

As you bring your finger down say "*tap*." Repeat several times, tapping the baby's head each time you say the word "*tap*." Remember, tap firmly but gently.

### Level 2: Words associated with motion
### 7) UP and 8) DOWN

You don't need to set aside a special time to teach baby *up* and *down*. Just remind yourself to say, "*up*" whenever you stand up from a couch, bed, or chair. Whenever you plan to sit down, simply say, "*down*" as you are sitting. Don't sit or stand quickly; there is no need to, and you might lose your balance.

• **Tip:** You don't have to say "*up*" or "*down*" every time you move, only when it is convenient for you.

### 9) SWAY

Stand with feet apart, about shoulder width. Move from side to side while you repeat the word, "*sway*."

Don't sway in places where you could strike your abdomen or arms, or in a position where you could lose your balance. "*Sway*" works really well in time with music.

### 10) ROCK

Sit with your hands on your knees. Rock back and forth, using a rhythm that is comfortable for you and repeat the word "*rock*." You can sit in a rocking chair to do this exercise if you choose.

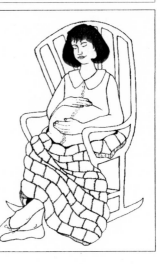

• **Tip:** Your practice with the Primary Words, "*sway*," "*rock*," "*drop*," and "*squeeze*" also helps prepare the baby for the birth process. We have some suggestions about using these words and the sensations they represent during the birth process. See **Labor and Delivery** section for more on this subject.

## Level 3: Words associated with sounds

Music and other rhythmical sounds sooth your baby (slow, repetitive sounds) or make your baby more alert and active (more rapid, changing sounds). We recommend that you learn to use quieting sounds on a regular basis at times when you would like your baby to sleep after she is born.

The goal in teaching the word *music* is to train your baby to associate the sound of the word with a variety of musical sounds. Soft and soothing music, without a lot of percussion, works best. After a while of working with music, you may find some selections that your baby seems to like. One kind of music may quiet your baby down, another may result in more activity. Keep notes for yourself about these preferences. They may be useful after your baby is born in helping to develop better sleeping patterns or comforting your baby when she is upset.

Preborn babies and infants respond favorably to classical music played at moderate volume levels. According to some research results, they especially seem to enjoy the music of Baroque and Classical era composers such as Bach, Handel, Pachelbel, Vivaldi, Haydn, Mozart, and Beethoven.

Popular or contemporary styles of music can also be pleasing for children to listen to, but generally babies do not respond favorably to very loud sounds of any kind. Loud rock music tends to irritate and agitate them, according to research findings by Dr. Thomas Verny, author of *The Secret Life of the Unborn Child*.

You can play music for your preborn by putting a tape recorder on your abdomen or by placing a small speaker on your abdomen. Another way you can play these musical selections is to use headphones that reach across your abdomen.

Select various kinds of music, and don't play them too loudly. More than 80 decibels applied to the uterine wall can be disturbing to the baby. You wouldn't want to place your ear near a running blender or a blaring music speaker for more than a few seconds. It's the same for your baby. It the sounds are too loud, the baby will be uncomfortable. Our experience indicates that rock concerts or very loud live or recorded dance music may be too loud for the baby. Please use common sense for this.

Remember the guidelines for levels of sound. If you can hear the tape recorder from about 15 feet away, it is loud enough. The idea is to get about 80 decibels to your baby through the mother's abdominal wall (a level that will not be too loud for the baby and yet loud enough to be distinguished from the other sounds inside the body, such as stomach sounds, heartbeat, etc. If you do not have good hearing your-self, we suggest you check these volume levels with a person who you know has normal hearing levels.

The following are sound levels of typical home sound sources at a distance of 12 inches:

a) 1/4 H.P. electric motor  60 decibels
b) medium size fan 70 decibels
c) normal listening T.V. 75 decibels
d) water running in tub  80 decibels
e) upright vacuum  93 decibels
f) kitchen blender  106 decibels

A useful thought for you to keep in mind is that New York City sub-way trains sometimes produce screeching sounds of up to 120 deci-bels. Some factories and offices also have very loud equipment sounds. Your baby is a captive audience, going wherever you go and hearing whatever you hear.

Do you want your baby to be more familiar with the sounds of the subway or the machinery at your place of work than with your own soothing voice or pleasing musical melodies? Remember this when you practice, but don't be afraid to let your voice be loud enough to project the sounds and vibrations so your baby can hear you and what you choose to play for him.

---

### 11) MUSIC

Locate the baby's head. Place a small, portable radio or tape cassette play-er on your abdomen near the baby's head. Say *"music."* Within two seconds, turn the radio or cassette player on. In this way, the baby will learn to connect the word *music* with the sound of music.

Repeat this several times. When you stop the music, you can say, *"not music"* to tell baby the music has stopped.

## Variation

Beginning at about the 8th month of your pregnancy, play musical selections for about 10-15 minutes. Repeat the same selection for about a week before changing to a new one. Playing this same music in the delivery room may help to calm your baby when she is being born.

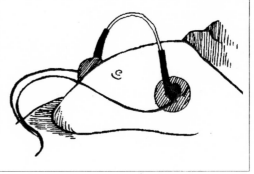

## 12) LOUD and 13) NOISE

The use of *loud* and *noise* can be helpful to protect your baby from becoming startled by dramatic changes in noise levels that we as adults have learned to ignore or accept. For example, your preborn may become startled by the sound of a chainsaw being turned on or firecrackers exploding. You can also say, *"loud"* or *"noise"* before slamming your car door closed.

## 12) LOUD

Place a radio or tape recorder near your abdomen. Set the music to the level that you normally use for the baby. Say, *"loud."* Pause one second. Turn up the volume for a few seconds. Then turn volume down to the normal setting. In this way your baby will be learning to anticipate sudden loud sounds.

• **Tip:** You can also use your own voice to do this exercise.

## 13) NOISE

Noise is best practiced when you are doing something that is loud and noisy such as vacuuming the floor. Say, *"noise."* Pause one second and then turn the vacuum on. Do your housework. Turn the vacuum off. Wait one second. Say, *"not noise."*

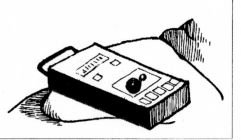

## Level 4: Words associated with mother's and baby's biological functions.

## 14) COUGH

Because you will most likely have to cough sometime during your pregnancy, you can help prepare your baby for the sudden, dramatic disturbance in his world by teaching him the word *cough.* Say, *"cough."* Within a second or two imitate the sound of a cough. Repeat.

## 15) SNEEZE

As soon as you finish sneezing, say, *"sneeze."* This may not be easy to do if there are other people around who would immediately say, *"Gesundheit"* or *"God Bless you."* So, we recommend you only practice the word *sneeze* when you are by yourself.

**16) HICCUP** *You may teach the word "hiccup" in two ways.*

## Variation 1
Say, *"hiccup."* Imitate the sound of a hiccup.

## Variation 2 (Baby's)
You could save this particular word for when you observe spasmodic twitching from the baby, which researchers believe to be a normal prenatal occurrence associated with fetal hiccups. When you observe the twitching, say *"hiccup"* loudly.

• **Tip:** Choose only one of the two hiccup exercises, because using both will be confusing to the baby.

---

**17) CRY**

Say, *"cry."* Follow immediately with the sound of crying.

*Cry* is best practiced as a pretend cry. If you have other children, they may be willing to share a cry with their preborn brother or sister. Ask your child if it would be alright if the baby could hear him or her cry for a short time. Say, *"cry,"* first and then bring the child close to your abdomen. Sometimes when you say to the crying child, *"That's fine. Thank you for letting your baby sister know what crying sounds like,"* your child may even stop crying. You can only use this strategy occasionally. It works best when the child is close to stopping the tears anyway, so you can prevent any resentment toward the baby. You should also feel comfortable sharing your own real cries with your baby. Perhaps, you can even tell him or her why you are crying and in that way soothe yourself.

---

**18) LAUGH**

Say, *"laugh."* Follow immediately with the sound of laughing.

You can pretend to laugh, but when something genuinely strikes you as funny, try to say the word *laugh* before or while you are laughing to let your baby know what is going on.

With any behavior such as laughing or crying that accompanies emotion, there may be chemical messengers that are reaching the baby through your bloodstream. So, let your baby in on what is occurring when it seems right to you.

## Level 5:  Words associated with vision
Your preborn should be ready to respond to this exercise after about the 35th week of pregnancy. We have had extensive experience in using light to stimulate babies in the womb, so we strongly recommend you strictly follow each step when doing this exercise.

## 19) LIGHT and 20) DARK

Locate the baby's head. Place a very bright light (a halogen flashlight, not a regular flashlight) in the lower part of the abdomen in the direction the baby is looking (this will be on the side opposite to the back). Turn the light on. Leave the light on for 3 seconds while you say, "*light*." Turn the light off. As you do so, say, "*dark*."

## Variation 1

You may use the words *on* and *off* for the light stimulus as an advanced lesson, such as "*light on*" and "*light off*."

• **Tip:** *Light* and *dark* works best in a darkened room where there is maximum contrast between dark and light.

*One afternoon one of our repeating Prenatal Classroom mothers who was pregnant with her second child brought along her 4-year old boy to a prenatal check-up. The mother and I reminisced about how she had used the Prenatal Classroom exercises during her first pregnancy. She reminded me that she had attended our prenatal class almost five years before.*

*I turned to the boy and asked him if he remembered when he was inside of his mommy. He said, 'Yes, I do.' I then asked if he could remember anything about being in there and he said, 'Yes, there was a light down there, and I didn't know where it was coming from.*

*I asked the mother if she had used the 'light' exercise in the class and afterwards. At first she didn't remember, but then suddenly she said, 'Yes!' She had learned it during the class and had used it about four or five times afterwards during the course of her pregnancy. She hadn't recalled doing it since the birth of her son and had never discussed the exercises with him.*

(Comment from Dr. Van de Carr that prenatal babies can see as well as remember)

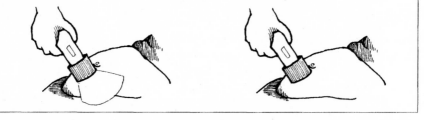

## Level 6: Words associated with temperature

You may want to add to the Primary Word List with words which describe stimuli you notice your baby responds to, like temperature. Some of our mothers have said that in late pregnancy when they drink cold water and repeat the word "*cold*," the baby responds.

Use the words *cold* and *hot* only late in pregnancy when baby is starting to press against Mom's stomach. Use these next two exercises when it is convenient and fits into your activities or when you are drinking something appropriate for teaching one of the words.

The stomach lies directly above the thin, distended wall of the uterus. These exercises are only effective in the last month of pregnancy when the uterus size is sufficiently large enough to elevate the stomach and provide wide areas of contact between baby and the stomach wall.

---

**21) COLD**

   Say, *"cold."* Drink something cold like a glass of ice water or lemonade. Say, *"cold, cold, cold"* about 60 seconds after you finish the drink.

---

**22) HOT**

   Say, *"hot."* Drink something hot like a cup of decaffeinated tea or coffee, or hot water with lemon. Say, *"hot, hot, hot"* about 60 seconds after you finish the drink. When you definitely have a warm sensation, repeat the word *"hot"* or *"warm"* several times, or *"not cold."*

---

## Level 7: Words that involve your baby's movements

   These words are only practiced when you feel the baby do them. They do not necessarily occur solely during any of your practice times. When you feel your baby kick, roll, or push (seems to stretch out in your womb), you can say the word that you feel best describes what your baby is doing. It is not necessary to do this every time you feel one of these sensations. Just do it when you feel like it.

---

**23) KICK** -say *"kick"* when you feel the baby kick.
**24) PUSH** -say *"push"* when you feel your baby stretching out and pressing against both sides of your abdomen.
**25) ROLL** -say *"roll"* when you feel a circular position change or turning of your baby.

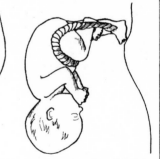

• **Tip:** You can add other words to the Primary Word List. Make sure they describe stimuli the baby can experience inside the womb and use them with the same stimulus each time.

---

## Level 8: Word to convey stopping of action
**26) NOT**

   You may say the word *"not"* with any of the words on this list to teach your baby that *"not"* means the absence or stopping of something. After you practice with a word by itself for a while, you could introduce the variation of *"not ......"* when you stop the stimulus. For example, you could say, *"not pat"* when you stop patting or *"not light"* when you turn off the flashlight. Adding *"not,"* however, should only follow after a period of at least 4 weeks of exposure to the Primary Word List.

# Primary Words Review Table

## Touch Words

PAT
RUB
SQUEEZE
SHAKE
STROKE
TAP

## Movement Words

UP
DOWN
SWAY
ROCK

## Sound Words

MUSIC
LOUD
NOISE

## Biological Words

COUGH
SNEEZE
HICCUP
CRY
LAUGH

## Vision Words

LIGHT
DARK

## Thermal Words

COLD
HOT

## Action Words Baby Makes

KICK
PUSH
ROLL

## Stopping of Action Word

NO

# Making Word Groups
## Advanced Version of Primary Word List
**Goal:** To begin grouping Primary Words into meaningful phrases. Grouping words can further your baby's pre-awareness of language in several ways:

**1)** The action (Primary Word) can become associated with a "do-er" (Ma Ma, Da Da, etc.). Your baby will become aware that a familiar sound such as "Ma Ma" is followed by another familiar sound (*"pat,"* *"rub,"* etc.). Example: *"Ma Ma pat baby."*

**2)** Grouping helps you differentiate body parts and teach the names of those parts to baby. Example: *"Da Da rub back."* or *"Da Da rub foot."*

**3)** Phrases present your baby with familiar sounds and sensations that are connected and form a sequence.

**4)** Present the rudimentary idea that simple things can build to form more interesting and complex concepts.

**5)** Present the parents with the concept that language naturally goes from simpler forms to greater complexity and specificity. Mom and Dad get used to using simple words that baby can understand and then build the words into more complex ideas.

## Materials needed: None

**When to begin:** You can start more advanced statements at about eight months (32 weeks), after working with the Primary Word List for three or four weeks.

**How often the exercise should be done:** As you become more proficient at the simple Primary Word List, you will start to add and build onto these word groups. They are part of the general session and do not need separate time.

These phrases are not a substitute for the Primary Words. By this time in your pregnancy you have practiced the Primary Words by themselves for three or more weeks. Use one practice time per day for the Primary Words by themselves and another for more advanced word groupings.

# Advanced Version of the Primary Word List

**Step 1:** Use the Primary Words *pat, rub, squeeze,* and *tap* in short sentences to help differentiate body parts. *Shake* and *stroke* will not work easily for this purpose.

    1) **PAT** Instead of saying only *"pat, pat, pat,"* as you pat the baby, you could say, "Ma Ma *pat bottom."* or "Ma Ma *pat head."*

    2) **RUB** As you teach the baby the word *"rub,"* say, "Ma Ma *rub back."*

    3) **SQUEEZE** When teaching *"squeeze,"* you could say, "Ma Ma *squeeze bottom."*

    4) **TAP** When teaching *"tap,"* say, "Ma Ma *tap head."* or "Ma Ma *tap bottom."*

## Variation 1

If someone else is talking to the baby, Dad for example, he would say, "Da Da *pat bottom."* Baby may be able to recognize Dad's deeper voice by 32 weeks or earlier.

## Variation 2

You can also try patting in time with mother's heartbeat. This is an advanced exercise to be used optionally. It combines three important sounds or feelings at once:

    A) the sound of the heartbeat
    B) the patting of the abdomen in time with the heartbeat
    C) the saying of *"pat, pat"* in time with the heartbeat.

This exercise can be done with father listening to mother's heartbeat and making the pats while mother says *"pat, pat"* in time with dad's hand. Or, mother can do the exercise by herself using a stethoscope (a minute is more than enough time for this exercise).

• **Tip:** Near the end of your pregnancy, you may begin to notice the baby moving differently to mother's, father's, sister's and/or brother's voices. Dr. Van de Carr has observed this change in response frequently enough to point it out to his patients. The change in reaction is a reminder that even though the baby in your womb cannot speak, he or she can have preference and is able to respond in a number of different ways. Just as our body language changes with different people, baby can react differently to each individual voice.

# Womb Stories and Songs

Womb stories and songs are a part of the Prenatal Classroom program that involves telling stories and singing to your preborn as a natural way of you two getting to know one another. You can start making up womb stories and songs using words from the Primary Word List. Your baby will be able to hear the words and feel their vibrations through your body.

Several of our colleagues have investigated the effects of reading stories, such as Dr. Seuss' *The Cat in the Hat*, to the preborn baby. They have reported increased intellectual and maturational development. In one study, a university researcher had a pregnant student repeatedly read a children's story out loud during her pregnancy. When her baby was born, he was tested for sound recognition, using the story that the baby's mother had read over and over again. The baby was also tested to see if he recognized the sounds of other stories. The baby definitely recognized the sounds of the one story that had been read by his mother.

We believe reading to your child before birth involves learning that is based upon the rhythm of the spoken word. Singing during pregnancy is another method of prenatal stimulation that enhances musical rhythm awareness in contrast to speech rhythms. The human brain has different centers that receive and process speech sounds and musical rhythms, so both of these activities stimulate different brain areas.

Remember, when you read or tell the baby stories, speak at more than your normal volume, enough so that someone standing 15 feet away could hear the words over the other noises in the room. We caution you from just going through the motions of reading to your baby. If you read in a monotone voice without interest in the material, you are conditioning baby to tune out rather than be excited by the spoken word.

If you have older children, position them near your abdomen and project your voice toward your abdomen while you read out loud. Or, position the children slightly below so you are speaking down toward your abdomen. The baby in your womb will hear and feel the rhythm of your "storytelling voice," so have a great time making the stories interesting by varying the pitch of your voice and the rhythms and rates at which you speak. For bedtime stories, slow the rhythm of your speech and see if your children become sleepy. If you don't have older children, you can:

**A)** Practice reading stories to children of friends, neighbors, and relatives. This is a great way to build up future babysitting credit, as well. Again, project your voice down toward your abdomen while you read and vary your pitch and rhythm.

**B)** Read to your husband, or have him read to you. You may even find some of these children's stories are more interesting than you thought. Or read poetry or other good sounding fiction aloud by yourself or to each other.

**C)** Read stories to the baby by yourself.

• **Tip:** If you don't enjoy reading aloud, try to find a way to make it more fun for yourself. If you can't, we suggest not trying to read aloud at all. We believe your baby can sense your moods, so why form a possible negative association toward listening to the written word?

## Womb Stories

In addition to reading aloud to your preborn, you can also make up short stories using words from the Primary Word List. Tell your baby the stories as you do the actions described.

Primary Words appear in boldface. Instructions appear in italics between parentheses.

*Example 1*

"Once upon a time Ma Ma was very happy. Ma Ma **rub** baby's back. (*rub baby's back*) **Rub** baby's back. Baby **laugh.** (*Mother should laugh*) Ma Ma said, '**Shake, shake, shake.**" (*shake your abdomen*) Oh yes, **shake, shake, shake.** (*shake your abdomen again*) and baby **laugh** again." (*Mother should laugh again*)

*Example 2*

"Once upon a time it was **dark.** (*start in a darkened room while relaxing*) Ma Ma **rock** baby. (*rock back and forth*) Ma Ma **sway** with baby. (*sway with baby*) Baby wake up. It is **light.** (*turn on flashlight for 3 seconds*) Ma Ma **pat** baby. (*pat your abdomen where baby's back is located*) Ma Ma **rub** baby's back." (*rub your abdomen where baby's back is located*)

Each time see how many different Primary Words you can use. While your baby becomes accustomed to hearing the sounds of the stories you tell, you are becoming a better storyteller. You will appreciate this skill after your baby is born when it comes time to lull your child to sleep.

## Womb Songs

Make up short songs using words from the Primary Word List. Sing these little songs as you repeat the actions, choosing whatever melody you want. As you sing, make the movements or actions that correspond to the Primary Words. It can be great fun making up your own songs and variations.

Primary Words appear in boldface. Instructions appear in italics between parentheses.

### Example 1

"La la la Ma Ma **pat** a bottom. (*pat your abdomen where baby's bottom is located*) la la la **pat** a head. (*pat your abdomen where baby's head is located*) la la la **rub** a back." (*rub your abdomen where baby's back is located*), etc.

One good tune to use is the "universal melody" that has many variations in cultures around the world but is best known in the United States as "*Ring Around the Rosie.*" Remember, as you sing, make the corresponding movements. As you sing the last line, "*Now all go down,*" sit down in a chair – do not actually fall. (You don't even have to sit down quickly.)

### Example 2

| | |
|---|---|
| Ma Ma pat the baby. | (*Ring Around the rosie*) |
| Ma Ma rub the baby. | (*Pocket full of posies*) |
| Sway | (*Ashes*) |
| and sway | (*Ashes*) |
| Now all go down | (*We all fall down*) |

### Variation

**Womb Dancing.** Try dancing while you sing the words "*up,*" "*sway,*" and "*rock.*" Try corresponding your movements to the words as you sing them. Again, please bear in mind that your body and center of gravity change during pregnancy, so use common sense when womb dancing.

Not every song you sing to baby has to be composed from the Primary Word List. You and your family can sing a favorite song or melody to your baby. We have had lots of parents do this and then later discover that the melody is comforting to the babies after birth and will lull them to sleep.

*With our first daughter, I sang her a folk song melody that I had liked from my childhood. I used to sing the melody with my head down close to my wife's belly. The song only lasted a minute or two, and it felt very good to me when I sang it. After our daughter was born I continued to sing the melody and she would listen, smile, close her eyes, and rest or go to sleep. It continues to be a beautiful experience for me, and*

*I still occasionally hum the song to her after telling her a bedtime story even though she is now over 8 years old.*

(Comment from a Prenatal Classroom father)

Keep song variations in the same order from session to session. Evidence suggests that baby can remember the sequence of what you do. So, if you start with a variation on "*Ring Around the Rosie*" and then go on dancing and singing a song, repeat that sequence in subsequent sessions.

# Teaching Numbers

**Goal:** To introduce baby to the concepts of numbers and counting in conjunction with some of the Primary Words.

**Materials needed:** None

**When to begin:** You should start using numbers in conjunction with Primary Words only after you have been working with variations of the Primary Word List, usually about the middle of the eighth month. By this time, you should have been working with the Primary Word for at least ten days.

Numbers are part of the general communication session. The procedure used is similar to what you will do in the other advanced activities. You will probably not want to use numbers higher than 3 or 4.

**How often the exercise should be done:** A special time is not necessary. Just include the numbers during some of your practice times.

INSTRUCTIONS

**Step 1:** You can begin teaching numbers by continuing to use the words the baby knows but adding a number.

**1) ONE** To teach your preborn baby the concept of *"one,"* modify a word or phrase you have already been using. For example, you have been using *"pat "* when you pat the baby's back. So say, *"one pat"* while giving baby a pat on the back, then stop and say something else, such as *"rub, rub, rub"* while rubbing baby's back, then say *"one pat"* again while giving baby a pat on the back. The idea is to use *"one pat"* when you pat the baby one time. Then go on to something else.

## Variation

Say "Ma Ma *one pat bottom*," and pat the baby's bottom once. Try this with other parts of baby's body.

**2) TWO** To teach the baby *"two,"* you would use the same stimulus twice. Say, *"two pat,"* and pat the baby's bottom twice.

## Variation

If father is talking to the baby, he should identify himself by saying, "Da Da *two pat bottom*."

**3) COUNTING**

"*One pat*" (pat one time) (pause)

"*Two pat*" (pat two times) (pause)

"*Three pat*" (pat three times) (pause)

"*Four pat*" (pat four times) (pause)

We suggest that you not simply say, "*One, two, three, four*" while omitting the word *"pat"* because this involves the use of the numbers as abstracts and will confuse the baby. He will not know if the sensation of being patted should be associated with the word *"pat"* or with the words *"one," "two," "three,"* or *"four."*

# The Xylophone Game

## Increasing Your Baby's Attention Span

Up to this point, you have been doing Prenatal Classroom exercises which are designed to make contact with your baby and give baby an opportunity to respond. These exercises have systematically stimulated your baby's developing senses – hearing, feeling, and perceiving light.

In this next part of the Prenatal Classroom program you will begin teaching baby to get used to waiting for something to happen. This is the beginning of what we call "paying attention." The game involves playing musical tones for your baby. We recommend using a tubular xylophone, but a guitar or piano are also easy to use.

Please be sure these instruments are in tune because we are also conditioning baby to be aware of exact tones and developing his sense of pitch. More specific suggestions for instruments can be found under the **Materials needed** heading.

Because your baby is now used to receiving consistent stimulation, he or she is developing a pre-awareness that sounds, touches, and even light can change and have meaning. This is not to say that your baby will be thinking, *"Oh, that's a pat, and that's a rub."* However, at some level your baby is becoming aware that there is a difference between a pat, a rub, and the other sensations you have introduced.

The Xylophone Game contains several levels of play, from very simple lessons to more complex games with different goals. We will describe five variations of increasing complexity, so you can select whichever fits your available time the best. As you become more practiced and familiar with what to do, you can move to more complex variations. After you have completed an exercise and move on to the next level, you do not need to repeat the earlier version except as an occasional review.

In its simplest form, the Xylophone Game, through repetition and association of notes and their names, (A, B, C, etc.) acquaints your baby with musical notes.

In its more advanced versions, the Xylophone Game can help develop your baby's ability to concentrate and to increase his or her attention span. Our research has shown us that at the point in development when you start the Xylophone Game (about 28 weeks) your baby's attention span may be less than two seconds. By adding to the time between saying the letter and striking the note, the Xylophone Game provides a repetitive exercise geared towards an increase in attention span.

Using the xylophone this way can also teach your baby that spoken sounds can be used to predict and describe future events. Your baby will be learning the time relationship between stimuli (tones made by the xylophone) and individual sounds of the first seven letters of the alphabet.

Just as we may "hear" the notes of a song that we know by heart, we believe that after a number of repetitions in which you say "A," (or any of the first seven letters), the baby can hear, even before you strike the note, the correct tone in his head.

Perhaps you are wondering if your baby can really learn to recognize tones. Our own research and that of many others seems to indicate that this is so.

One of our colleagues, Dr. Robert Fried of Hunter College in New York, conducted an experiment which showed that 14-day old chicken embryos could learn musical notes and respond to them. After the chicks were hatched, they still responded to the tones they had learned while still in the egg.

Along similar lines, and as we noted earlier in the section entitled **Heartbeats and Drum Rhythms,** some babies exposed to symphonic musical selections while in the womb were able to play notes on a piano and could pick out simple melodies several months to two years after birth.

During the first week of playing the Xylophone Game with your baby, you are working to establish an association between the letter of the musical note, such as "A," and the corresponding tone played on the xylophone. As you pair the sound of the letter "A" with the sound of the corresponding note, your baby will begin to expect that combination. He or she is making an association between the two.

You begin to increase your baby's attention span the second week by pausing for an additional second between saying the name of the note and striking the corresponding tone. Your pause between the name of the note and the tone will be another second longer during the third week and so on.

Each time you increase the length of your pauses, you are increasing baby's attention span. She has to wait just a little longer each week to hear the expected tone. We believe that you can increase your preborn's attention span up to a maximum of 5 seconds before her attention turns elsewhere.

Keep teaching the Primary Word List, drum patterns, musical stimulations, and other games you have already practiced with your baby. The use of musical tones to develop your baby's attention span will become a part of the lesson plan.

At this point in your reading, you may be wondering how many exercises you must fit into a session and how long each session should run. Many of our parents tend to pick out certain exercises that seem to fit them best. Enjoy yourself and remember, five to ten minutes per session seems to work well.

• **Tip:** If you have more time, you may wish to use some of the more advanced levels of the Xylophone Game. Most parents seem to enjoy playing these games with their baby.

## The Xylophone Game

**Goal:** To increase your baby's attention span. An additional goal is to teach exact tones and accurate pitch.

**Materials needed:** A small, tonally accurate, tubular or metal strip xylophone and a hollow tube or megaphone. You may use other tuned musical instruments such as a toy piano, electric organ, a tuned guitar, or a pitch pipe. However, most other instruments are not as practical, are not as accurate in pitch, don't sound as good, and are not as easy to carry as a small xylophone. A seven-note xylophone is more portable and easier to use than a larger one.

You will notice the notes on the xylophone are arranged from low to high. Try to obtain a xylophone upon which the first note is C, then D, then E, F, G, A, and B. Practice with the xylophone so you can strike the notes in any sequence. You don't have to practice in alphabetical order or by using a solely ascending or descending scale. In fact, it is better if you vary the sequence each time. We want baby to learn that notes can occur in many different orders, not just from low to high or high to low.

**When to begin:** Any time after the seventh month (28 weeks) of pregnancy, or after at least ten days of practice with the Primary Word List.

**How often the exercise should be done:** This exercise is part of the general session, and you do not need to set aside additional or separate time for it. You may wish to include it in only one of the two daily stimulation sessions.

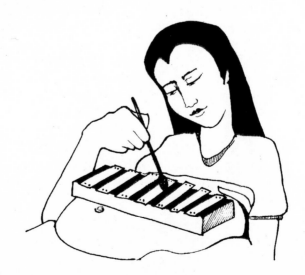

# First Level Xylophone Exercise

INSTRUCTIONS

Baby becomes acquainted with the musical notes. This is done by repetition and association between the name of the note and the sound of the note. In general, your baby will prefer higher tones over lower tones. For this reason start with the upper A on your xylophone. As you progress move to B and then to C and so on. Use all of the notes when you first introduce this exercise.

**Step 1:** Locate the baby's head. Place the xylophone (or other musical instrument you will be using) directly on your abdomen, over the position of the baby's head. It is best if you can remove any extra clothing and have the xylophone in direct contact with the skin. This way the sound of the xylophone will not be muffled.

**Step 2:** Say the letter "A." Pause 1 second.

**Step 3:** Strike the note A on the xylophone. Pause 3 seconds. (You are beginning to teach your baby to expect a tone following the spoken word.)

**Step 4:** Repeat the letter "A." Pause 1 second.

**Step 5:** Strike the note A again. Pause 3 seconds.

**Step 6:** Repeat steps 1 through 5 for the next note, B. Follow steps 1 through 5 for each note.

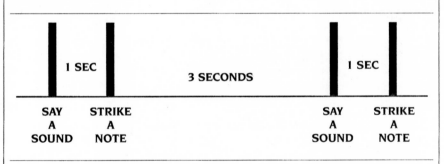

You can do as many notes as you feel like doing during each learning session. We believe three different notes are good to start with, after you have introduced baby to all of the notes. There is not a need to do all of the notes on the xylophone each time you practice. Do this basic exercise for two weeks.

• **Tip:** Don't say or sing anything else during the Xylophone Game. Other words or notes will confuse the baby about the relationship between the letters you are saying and the notes you are striking. If you are knowledgeable in music theory, you may wish to pick notes that make chord patterns for some of the repetitions later in your practice. You may also want to tap your foot while counting the beats as a musician would do to keep time. Your baby will feel the beats when you do this.

# Second Level Xylophone Exercise

The purpose here is to build your baby's concentration and expand his or her attention span by adding time between saying the letter and striking the note.

Use same exercise as level 1, but increase pause between saying the letter and striking the note to 2 seconds. The pause between each pairing of note and tone will be 2 seconds plus 2 seconds= 4 seconds.

**Step 1:** Locate the baby's head. Place the xylophone on your abdomen near where the baby's head is located.

**Step 2:** Say the letter "A." Pause 2 seconds.

**Step 3:** Strike the note A on the xylophone. Pause 4 seconds.

**Step 4:** Repeat the letter "A." Pause 2 seconds.

**Step 5:** Strike the note A again. Pause 4 seconds.

**Step 6:** Follow steps 2 through 5 for the next note, B. Follow steps 2 through 5 for each note.

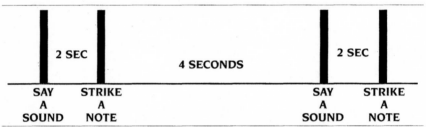

When pauses between saying the note and striking the note are longer than 4 seconds, this exercise will start to take a little more time. So, proceed with the longer pauses only when you have the time. Again, do not exceed 5-second pauses between saying and playing the notes.

## Variation 1

In this version, you are going to repeat the letter of the note twice and then hit the note twice.

## Variation 2

Repeat the letter of the note three times, then hit the note three times.

## Variation 3

**Elementary Categorization** (advanced & optional). This is a very advanced version in which you'll combine two or three notes, A, B, and C to make patterns, such as AB, AC, BC, ABC, CAB, CCB, etc.). Say the letters one after another with little pause. Then wait two seconds and strike the corresponding notes. This variation is teaching your baby to recognize groupings at a rudimentary level. Try this variation only after you have been doing the previous exercises for one month.

• **Tip:** Towards the end of your pregnancy, go back to the simplest forms of the exercises for some practice sessions. Your preborn will enjoy the familiar words and tones.

# The Secondary Word List

From your work so far your baby has learned that words are important and have meaning in his or her world. In the last month (or three weeks) of pregnancy, you can further expand baby's awareness of the external world by using the words of the Secondary Word List. These are words for things that the baby cannot experience within the uterus. The words on this list describe things that will be important to the baby in the first four months of life and may begin to familiarize baby with the sounds of words he or she will hear after birth.

In addition to teaching your baby the sounds of the words, you are starting to pass on your own speech patterns and dialect. Baby will come to recognize these along with the tone of your voice. Even in the first days after birth elements of your speech patterns can be detected in baby's cries and coos.

*The work of Henry Truby shows that the earliest cry spectrographs of very premature fetuses already contain some of the speech characteristics seen in their mothers' spectrographs. Add to this the fact that newborns of mute mothers (or deaf newborns) do not cry, or cry strangely at birth indicates what happens when we are deprived of speech in utero.*

(Dr. David Chamberlain, author of Babies Remember Birth)

# The Secondary Word List

1) Love
2) Kiss
3) Sleep
4) Talk
5) You
6) Milk
7) Wet
8) Dry
9) Diaper (*or other word for diaper that you will be using*)
10) Ba Ba (*for milk bottle*)
11) Ma Ma Ba Ba (*milk from breast*)
12) Go
13) Come back
14) Burp
15) Apple juice
16) Grandma
17) Grandpa
18) Eye
19) Nose
20) Mouth
21) Arm
22) Leg
23) Finger
24) Ear
25) Tongue
26) Powder
27) Water
28) Brother
29) Sister
30) Throw up
31) Oh Oh, Pu Pu, or Ka Ka (*diaper change*)
32) Yawn
33) Ice cream
34) Cereal

## The Secondary Word List

**Goal:** The purpose of the Secondary Word List is to familiarize your baby with these words, so that after he or she is born, you can begin to connect these words with the objects they represent. You, as the teacher, are also developing a habit of saying the words clearly to your baby and thinking about the items that you use every day.

**When to begin:** You can start this learning game in the 34th week of your pregnancy, and you will continue it after birth. Once the baby is born, the teaching will consist of straightforward statements such as, *"This is your nose." "This is your mouth." "This is your diaper."*

**How often the exercise should be done:** The Secondary Word List will become part of your regular communication sessions. You do not need to set aside a separate time to do these.

### *The Secondary Word List*

---
INSTRUCTIONS

Repeat the words clearly toward the end of the learning session. It may be convenient to shorten the list depending on your available time. Pick those words that you are likely to use soon after the birth of your baby.

---

# Infant Speak
## (Optional)

The ten words listed in this section comprise what we call Infant Speak. They should not be thought of as "baby talk." They were designed to be introduced before the baby is born and used by both parents and baby after birth.

Infant Speak is a unique part of the Prenatal Classroom program. These basic word tools follow universal speech patterns based on monosyllabic, repetitive sounds used by infants in most cultures. Infant Speak words are designed to allow the baby to have an early verbal interaction with his or her environment. This allows baby to express emotions on a verbal level as well as on a physical level which, in turn increases her confidence in expressing her own needs and feelings.

When a baby first begins to speak, the sounds she makes are frequently difficult for adults to understand. So, we label them as "babble" and don't pay attention to what baby is trying to say. By reinforcing baby's natural tendency to use sounds together, we make the message clearer for adults to understand. For example, a baby saying, "B*a*" might be misunderstood, but a clearly spoken "B*a* B*a*" means baby is hungry.

97

Your baby will even come to know when Infant Speak words are pronounced incorrectly.

*One of our Prenatal Classroom babies, (who while in the womb had listened repeatedly to Infant Speak words played on a tape recorder during the last month of pregnancy), shortly after birth listened attentively and smiled when her mother said the Infant Speak words. When her grandmother whose first language was not English, mispronounced these words, she would immediately fret or cry.*

(Comment from Dr. Van de Carr about baby's memory of speech patterns)

Infants will communicate with you in any way they can. They most commonly do this by crying. But infants repetitively stimulated in the womb will try to use that stimuli to tell you what their needs are. A friend of Dr. Van de Carr's discovered after the birth of his baby that the infant was using an odd form of communication he had assimilated while still in his mother's womb. Dr. Van de Carr explains:

*A colleague of mine who is a psychologist and internationally known lecturer related a personal experience while sitting at lunch one day. He and his wife had a habit during her pregnancy of sitting in a swing at their home at the end of the day. They would rock back and forth while holding hands and listening to the recordings of whale calls and songs. After the baby was born, both father and mother were actively involved in caring for the baby. On one occasion when the father was babysitting, he decided to reprogram the message on his answering machine. While doing this, the baby had awakened and started to cry. My colleague did not respond immediately. Then he became aware that the baby's cry had somehow changed. It sounded strange but at the same time familiar. The cry was repeated over and over. Later, when he had taken care of his baby's needs, he returned to the answering machine and played the message he had just recorded. There in the background of the recording but still clear was the sound of a whale calling over and over.*

Here we see how the mother, who was feeling pleasure rocking back and forth in the swing, and emotionally supported by her husband, was sending biological messages of contentment to the baby. The baby itself was sensing his mother's gentle rocking motions and could hear the cry of the calling whales. This was repeated over and over during pregnancy, just like the stimuli you will be presenting to your baby in the Prenatal Classroom exercises.

The baby's whale call message is clear. He was saying, "Come Da Da. Come pick me up and rock me."

Because your baby can learn, remember, and recreate sounds and words, you should be careful about what you say in his or her presence. Be especially careful not to say any words that you don't want to hear coming from your child's mouth later.

*Here is another example of what can happen when you don't pay attention to the words that you use with your baby. One mother in my practice who had stimulated her preborn baby occasionally muttered, "Yuk" after his birth when she had to change a diaper for her baby. By the time the baby was 3 months old he would say, "Yuk, yuk, yuk" when he needed his diaper changed. What would you prefer to hear your baby saying?*

(Comment from Dr. Van de Carr about the effects of early language stimulation)

## Infant Speak Word List

1) Ma Ma (*mother*)
2) Da Da (*father*)
3) Ba Ba (*a feeding from breast or bottle*)
4) Din Din (*food other than milk*)
5) Oh Oh, Pu Pu, or Ka Ka (*diaper change*)
6) No No (*no*)
7) Eh Eh (*come to me*)
8) Ni Ni (*time to sleep*)
9) Hi Hi (*greeting*)
10) Bye Bye (*leaving or separation*)

**Goal:** Infant Speak consists of words made from simple repetitive sounds, which allow the 1 to 12-month old infant the possibility of greater interaction with and control of his or her environment.

**When to begin:** If you wish, you may start Infant Speak during the last month of your pregnancy. It is optional. After your baby is born, try the Infant Speak words. If your baby likes them, continue to use them. Perhaps your baby will prefer another word for sleep or food. If so, use that. We have found that these words are easy for most parents to use, and most babies like them.

**How often the exercise should be done:** Infant Speak should be presented to the baby with extra stimulation sessions which are devoted to these words only. One or two of these extra sessions should be done each day. Repeat the list five times during the session. There is no particular time of day that is best, and you should be guided by your schedule. If you would like, you can record the Infant Speak words and the Secondary Words you want to use on a tape recorder and play them for the baby once a day.

# Infant Speak

# Examples of Prenatal Classroom Learning Sessions at Different Stages of Your Pregnancy

We provide these guidelines to give you typical amounts of time and sequences for using the Prenatal Classroom program exercises. We feel it is most important that you do the exercises in a way that you feel good while doing them. Once you are familiar with the exercises you will discover how easy it is to find the few moments each day to practice.

## First Phase Exercises (Getting Your Preborn's Attention)
*18-28 Weeks*

Generally two sessions per day. One session with Dad or helpers if possible. Plan the session about 30 minutes to 2 1/2 hours after mother eats so the preborn will be alert. Learning sessions during the First Phase generally last for one to five minutes.

**a)** 18-22 weeks: Basic Rhythms with 1/2 second between beats.

**b)** 20-24 weeks: Kick Game. You can also play the Kick Game at any other time when your preborn is active and kicking. (During your sessions, pause for about 2 minutes between the Basic Rhythms and the Kick Game or do the activities at different times.)

**c)** 24-28 weeks: Advanced versions of the Kick Game.

## Second Phase Exercises (First Words and Sensory Stimulation)
*27 Weeks and Up to Birth*

Generally two sessions per day. One session with Dad or helpers if possible. Plan the session about 30 minutes to 2 1/2 hours after mother eats so the preborn will be alert. Learning sessions during the Second Phase generally last 5 to 10 minutes.

**a)** Continue responding to kicks when they occur and use the Basic Rhythms three to four times per week.

**b)** 27th week on: Practice finding your baby's position. Practice for at least one week. As your baby develops it will become easier for you to figure out his or her position. It is best to coordinate your practice with a planned visit to your obstetrician, family practice physician, midwife, or other healthcare provider so you can check on finding your baby's head, back, and feet.

**c)** 28th week on: Start out your sessions with the Primary Words and use them several times per day. Practice using the main Primary Words in your stimulation sessions for several weeks. You can then add some of the other Primary Words and continue to practice up until birth.

**d)** After several weeks of using the Primary Words, begin to add womb stories and womb melodies after your Primary Word practice.

By this time you are becoming familiar with developing a good learning session routine. In some instances you will discover the activities and exercises that your preborn seems to prefer. It is important that you remain attentive to your baby and have fun while doing the sessions. It is better to miss a session than to feel hurried or distracted while doing the activities. We have taken care to modify the sessions so they are enjoyable and do not take up a lot of time.

## Third Phase Exercises:
## (Building Attention Spans and Words for the Outside World)
*28 Weeks to Birth*

In addition to the two regular sessions per day you may want to add a 10 minute music session at times when you think your preborn is less active or around 9 or 10 p.m. to help reinforce a positive sleep pattern after birth. Use some of the musical selections found in Appendix B. It is important for you to get some rest during these music sessions too. Music time is also a very good time for you to practice your hand warming and stress release exercises.

**a)** Continue with the Primary Words, womb melodies, and songs

**b)** 28th Week – Xylophone Game

**c)** 30th Week – Pre-Awareness of Numbers exercises

**d)** 31st Week – Infant Speak

**e)** 32nd Week – Secondary Words

After about a week of practice, add a new lesson to the session. These later sessions will last about 10 minutes. You don't need to do every activity during every session. As your preborn's teacher, you can vary the activities and select which ones to do depending on the level of activity of your preborn at the time, how you feel, and who is helping.

## Preparation For a Baby-Oriented Birth, Bringing Your Baby Home From the Hospital, and Introducing Your Baby to His or Her New Home

*35th Week to Birth*

Start reviewing the birth preparations by the beginning of your 9th month of pregnancy.

Continue with two to three learning sessions each day. Avoid, if possible, the hurried feeling that you have to get everything ready yourself. By doing the Prenatal Classroom exercises you have probably figured out that after your baby is born, you get a second chance to get acquainted all over again. *So why hurry?*

# PART IV
## *Giving Birth*

# Preparing For Your Baby's Birth

During the last few weeks of pregnancy you may notice a number of lazy periods where you feel more interested in daydreaming than anything else. These periods are associated with an increase in the amount of natural endorphins that are now being produced in your body. Endorphins are what produces the "runner's high" and are the body's natural pain suppressants. This means your body is getting ready to help you control pain during the birth process.

We recommend two ways to help this process work for you as much as possible.

**1)** Don't leave any large, unfinished projects that need to be done during the ninth month of pregnancy. We would like you to be on a regular schedule without extra demands during the ninth month. In this way, you will have time to notice and enjoy these natural relaxation periods and they will help to build your energy reserves for the birth process.

**2)** During the relaxation periods, picture yourself easily taking care of what you need to prepare for a good birth. Research has shown that thinking positively and imagining good results helps reduce anxiety and pain. It also tends to reduce complications during medical procedures. Finish the series of images by picturing yourself at home with your new baby and other family members around you. Some of our mothers have reported that during these periods they can actually feel themselves holding their baby, starting to nurse, or introducing baby to his or her new home.

## Music at the Birth

One of the most exciting times in your life can be what we call *Student Graduation* i.e., the process of labor and delivery. Because you may be anxious about getting to the ceremonies on time, keep everything you will need for your hospital stay in one place, ready to go. As your expected delivery date approaches, put your music exercise materials (music box, small tape recorder, xylophone, etc.) into the bag or suitcase you are planning to take with you to the hospital after you have finished using them.

We recommend that you prepare your "birth kit" about two weeks before your due date. Some parents also feel better making a trial run to practice getting everything (and everyone) into the car and driving to the hospital. If you do this, time yourself beginning from when you decide to leave to your arrival at the hospital. Then add 5 to 10 minutes for the unexpected.

Familiar music and words are reassuring to newborns, not only during the birth process but after birth as well. Nurses in the maternity ward tell of babies who will settle down when familiar music is played to them after all other attempts to calm them have failed. Another benefit is that by concentrating on your conversation with the baby, and on what the baby is hearing and feeling, you will find that your time in labor passes more quickly and easily.

*I don't know who enjoyed the music more, my husband, myself, or our little girl. We stayed overnight at the hospital for two days and listened to the three tapes we had used during my pregnancy. It was quiet, peaceful, and a great way to get to know our baby.*

(Comment from a Prenatal Classroom mother)

At many hospitals, tape recorders playing soothing music and video cameras capturing the event are welcomed in delivery suites. However, it is best to talk to your doctor and the nursing staff beforehand if you want to use either of these during the birth of your baby. Most birthing staffs will want to support you in anything that makes you feel comfortable, as long as it doesn't interrupt the necessary medical routine.

You will have to decide whether or not you want to tell the staff that you have been playing the music for the baby as well as for yourself. The same issue is also true for using the Primary Words during delivery. If your doctor and birthing staff are supportive, they will know that anything that you do to stay alert and attentive to the birthing process will help things go smoothly and will help keep you going if you get tired. If for some reason the birthing staff or doctor is not supportive (or can't be because of other medical reasons), just bear in mind that by having used Prenatal Classroom materials during pregnancy and by going to your birth preparation classes, you are well prepared and ready to let your baby come into the world.

## Exercises for a Baby-Oriented Birth

In contrast to most birth preparation methods which are "birth-oriented," we believe that it is preferable to focus more attention on the well-being of the baby. We call this approach a "baby-oriented" birth preparation.

The goal of a baby-oriented birth is to give mother's natural instinct to protect her baby more of a role in the birth. In this way, there can be natural suppression of pain and discomfort because the mother's attention is on the baby.

In a baby-oriented birth, the mother uses breathing, visualization, and other methods of support taught in birthing programs. Mother (and father or helper) attends to baby's progress toward birth while breathing to a coach's count and resting between the waves of a contraction-expansion.

Each of the prenatal stimulation exercises and activities you have already practiced can be used during a baby-oriented birth. Naturally, it they don't seem right, don't use them.

None of these exercises are meant to be used all the time during birth. Mothers will change them, shift from one to another and use other methods that give the most relief and comfort.

## Exercises for a Baby-Oriented Birth

**Goal:** To allow optimum strength and flexibility during delivery, to provide conditioning, and to help speed recovery after birth. These exercises also help you release the pain of contractions during labor.

**Materials needed:** None

**When to begin:** Start practicing these exercises in the last month of pregnancy.

**How often the exercise should be done:** Practice the exercises twice a week for short periods of time.

# Exercises for a Baby-Oriented Birth

**1) Squeeze breathing**

This first exercise teaches you how to breath during labor. Breathe in deeply through your nose. As you release the breath through your mouth, say the word, *"squeeeeeeeeeeeeeeeeeeeze"* long and slow. Each time a contraction comes during labor, you will breathe in deeply and release the contraction as you release your breath while saying, *"squeeeeeeeeeeeeeeeeeeeeze."* Loudness is not important here. Just concentrate on turning your blow into the word and letting out the discomfort each time you exhale.

In communication sessions you will use the word *"squeeze"* when not having contractions. In labor, however, we suggest that you use it only when you're having contractions.

**2) Standing and Releasing**

This exercise should be done during the first stage of labor. The goal here is to use an active breath release with words that you have practiced with your baby. This makes the first part of labor less uncomfortable and reassures your baby. As contractions begin, stand and stick out your abdomen as much as you can, allowing the position of the baby to move forward and become better aligned with the birth canal. Say, *"This is a squeeze, baby,"* Then say, *"squeeze"* again while slowly blowing out your breath.

**3) Birthing Sway**

This may be done in a standing position. While placing your hands on both sides of your abdomen, stick out your abdomen as much as you can. Sway slightly from side to side, allowing your abdomen to move to and fro. Inhale deeply through your nose. As you exhale and while you are still swaying, say the phrase, *"Sway, sway the pain away."* Say, *"sway, sway"* in a slightly louder voice and *"the pain away"* in a softer voice as you release the last part of your breath.

**Rocking and Releasing**

The goal of this exercise is to provide a relaxing release of pain during the first stage of labor when standing becomes uncomfortable. The second part of the exercise should be used during the transition to the second stage of labor.

First, practice rocking while sitting in a chair or on a firm bed, with your legs apart and your hands on the outside of your legs under the knees. An alternative position is to sit backwards on the chair so your legs are apart, your arms are supported by the top of the chair back, and your head rests on your arms.

Later, you will release two deep breaths and practice pulling up on your hands below the knees as you rock. Let the first two breaths turn into the word *"rock"* as you rock. Inhale again, but hold the third breath and think the word *"push"* before slowly exhaling.

Practice the three-breath cycle for 2 to 3 minutes and then relax.

## Good Blood Flow to the Uterus

The best position for allowing optimum blood flow to the uterus is for you to lay down turned to your left side with your head and shoulders supported and slightly elevated by a pillow. This will increase blood flow to the baby and is the recommended position for you to assume between contractions if you are lying down.

Remember that breathing too deeply for long periods of time may cause you to hyperventilate. The symptoms of hyperventilation include sweating and tingling or numbness in the hands. This condition can actually decrease the blood flow to the baby as arteries that supply blood to the placenta become constricted. To avoid this, limit your deepest breathing to the times when you are having active uterine contractions in labor and to relatively short periods of time during your practice sessions.

## Squatting or Lying Down for Delivery

Squatting during birth has some advantages in that gravity is helping the baby progress through the birth canal. There is also a potential psychological advantage in that the mother is very much in charge of the delivery in this position. However, in standard medical practice many mothers feel considerable discomfort squatting for the periods of time that are required for delivery (this is another reason to stay in good physical shape during your pregnancy). If it is comfortable for you, you can assume a squatting position just about anywhere, even on a hospital bed. Your doctor or midwife will be able to support you and give you advice about how to proceed should you consider delivering the baby this way.

## Contractions and Expansions

Many women fear contractions. They may have heard well-meaning but nonetheless intimidating stories from their mothers or friends about the pain associated with contractions.

It may be useful for you to know that what is called a contraction is really a squeezing of the uterus and its surrounding muscles, which acts to slowly send the baby down the birth canal until the moment of birth occurs. At the same time, the cervix (opening of the womb where the baby's head will emerge) is expanding. Each contraction of the uterus is also helping the cervix expand.

We recommend you make the connection in your mind that each contraction of your uterus is leading to an expansion of your cervix. This way of thinking allows you to picture each contraction ending with an expansion. You can also use mental imagery to visualize your cervix starting to open. By using this process, many women lessen the amount of muscle tightening accompanying contractions, thus reducing the amount of pain.

## Eating Close to Your Expected Delivery Time

When you become aware of going into the early stages of labor, don't eat a large meal. Some women feel that they will need to eat to have energy. In fact, if you eat a large meal the pressures of the early stages of delivery and the fullness of your stomach may increase your discomfort during labor. Large meals will also divert blood to the intestinal tract and may result in uncomfortable feelings, nausea, or vomiting. It also may be dangerous to eat a large meal if an anesthetic is needed.

# Labor and Delivery

It is important for you to realize that this is *your* birth process, and it is not necessary to use any of the Prenatal Classroom exercises during the birth if doing so doesn't seem right to you, if you need to conserve your energy, or if you need to express your feelings in other ways. You will have more than enough time to continue with what you have learned in the program after your baby is born.

## Prenatal Classroom in the Delivery Room

**Goal:** Using the learning games you have been playing for the past several months during labor will provide a reassuring environment of familiar stimuli to help your baby through what can otherwise be an alarming experience. By practicing contact and communication, you and your baby have become used to working together and responding to one another. This will help you both during labor and delivery.

**Materials needed:** This depends upon the exercise you choose. We suggest you choose exercises that don't require too many extra materials at this time. You'll already have to keep track of a tape recorder, if you have chosen to play music during labor and delivery.

**When to begin:** You may communicate with the baby during labor and delivery, just as you did at home before the baby was born.

**How often the exercise should done:** When possible, the baby should be patted, rubbed, and reassured in the intervals between contractions and your breathing exercises.

# Communicating With Your Baby During the Birth Process

**Step 1:** Talk directly to the baby, using *pat, rub, squeeze, sway,* and *rock* as you have been during the learning games and stimulation exercises. Your partner should place his cheek against your abdomen to talk with the baby in a reassuring manner.

Although at first it may be embarrassing or awkward to talk to the baby in the hospital setting, both you and your partner will soon get over these feelings if the situation seems right for you. You will most likely find that the nursing staff will respect your wishes and help you in every way possible.

If you are having a home delivery, or couldn't make it to the hospital on time, use what you have practiced to make the delivery as safe and easy as possible for you and the baby.

During delivery there can be times when mother doesn't want to be touched or needs to focus on her breathing or mental imagery to keep her mind off the pain.

## Variation 1

In addition to talking with the baby, your music source (music box or cassette tape player) can be placed on a nearby table or nightstand or even directly on your abdomen over the location of the baby's head and played between or during contractions and/or be available to be played for your baby after birth. Playing the music gives baby a soothing and familiar sound to listen to during the actual birth. Remember, music can also be helpful to you if it seems right.

## Variation 2

During some of the contractions, tell the baby, *"This is a squeeze."* This connects the sensation of labor with the baby's past experiences, with the word *"squeeze,"* and the feeling of being squeezed.

## Variation 3

If you are having a medicated delivery, or regional block anesthesia, there will be some differences in what you can expect. Although there probably will be some special monitoring attachments on your abdomen, your partner should be able to place his hand or head between them. If not, ask the nursing staff if it is possible to adjust the placement of the attachments, so that you can communicate with your baby.

## Variation 4

If you need to have a caesarean delivery, you can still use The Prenatal exercises you have practiced with your baby. You may have to wait until the necessary post-operative is completed before you again focus on your baby.

**Step 2:** If the delivery room at the hospital is different from the labor room, your music source can be taken into the delivery room and placed nearby or on your abdomen under the sterile drapes. Make sure if you do this that your husband, partner, or birth coach is responsible for the tape recorder or music box so it doesn't get left in the delivery room. Also tell the birthing staff so they know what to expect.

**Step 3:** After birth, we recommend you keep the baby with you for an hour or so, if it is possible. Hold your baby next to your body.

Even though you use up a lot of energy during the birthing process, we have seen time and time again women who have taken little or no medication to control pain experience a sudden surge of positive energy as soon as the baby is born. We believe this may be due to the body's chemical release of energy at birth that is nature's way of giving you the power to say, "Hello" and see, touch, and smell your new baby. (It is interesting to see how often pictures taken shortly after birth show a bright and energetic mother and a drained and pale father. It is usually a good thing for Dad to get a bit of rest after the delivery.)

Make eye contact with your baby (about 8 to 12 inches away) if you feel up to it. This will seem like the natural distance for you, and it is the distance at which your newborn's eyes can focus.

Nuzzle and smell your baby's head. This is a natural response of many animals, and we believe it is significant to positive bonding. Don't use unusual perfumes or shampoos prior to labor. Your baby should learn how you normally smell.

When your baby feels comfortable with you, he or she may try to nurse or sleep for a while with you.

Remember, depending upon the duration of your labor, the types of medication you received, and the conditions of your delivery, your baby may simply be too tired to respond to you as he or she might after some rest.

**Step 4:** When you are holding baby in your arms in the delivery room, repeat phrases from stimulation sessions to reassure him or her with familiar sounds. When the baby is placed in your arms, repeat the familiar phrases, "Hi, *this is Ma Ma. Pat, pat, pat.*" And, "*Ma Ma rub, rub, rub you.*" All the while pat or rub the baby's back. Similarly, your partner should soothe, pat, and rub the baby when his turn to hold the baby comes. Your baby will be looking at you, listening to your voice and will feel very happy to be with you.

# Congratulations!

# Delivery Stories

*She came out with a smile.*

(A spontaneous remark from an experienced midwife about a baby born while music that had been used prenatally was playing)

*I can always tell if it is one of Dr. Van de Carr's Pat, Pat, Rub, Rub babies. They always seem so alert and hardly cry at all.*

(Comment from a hospital nursery nurse when interviewed for a national television program about our prenatal stimulation program)

*I was called by a maternity nurse who in an excited voice stated that the baby's heartbeat was very rapid ( 210 beats per minute, a sign of fetal distress) and that she wanted to call her supervisor to start making arrangements for a Caesarean section for my patient. I knew that this patient and her husband had used the Prenatal Classroom exercises during their pregnancy. I went to the labor room and saw that the baby's head was barely visible in the vaginal opening. The nurse was attempting to help the delivery by massaging the muscles of the vagina. However, her fingers had been touching the baby's head. I told her to move her fingers away from touching the baby's head because this might be causing the rapid heartbeat. During the next minute or so the baby's heartbeat slowed down to a normal rate and stayed there for several minutes. I assured the mother that she wouldn't need a Caesarean and that she should prepare for letting the baby come when he was ready. In the meantime, I asked the nurse to touch the baby's head again. The heart rate went up to the same high rate as before. This time I asked the father who was also there to pat his wife's abdomen where the baby's back was located and to say in a soothing voice, "Pat, pat, pat. Da Da is here. It is OK." I told him to keep on repeating this. Even though the nurse was still touching the baby's head the heart rate went down to a normal rate, and a Caesarean section was averted. When this baby was born, he responded to his father's voice by moving his eyes toward his father.*

(Comment from Dr. Van de Carr on the dramatic effect of prenatal communication during labor.)

• **Tip:** Remember, on occasion the demands of good medical practice may interfere with plans for communication with the baby. Although disappointing, this is only a temporary postponement, and you can plan to resume communication after the baby is born, or whenever the baby's and mother's health permit.

## Bonding with Your Baby

Widespread research has shown that babies who were left on their mother's breast or abdomen for a minimum of one hour after birth had significantly better acceptance of breast feeding than babies who were taken from their mothers less than an hour after birth.

These new findings are consistent with what we have long advocated and practiced with parents who choose to participate in the Prenatal Classroom. Naturally, we are pleased our medical colleagues have come to the same conclusion through their own research. Prenatal Classroom mothers and fathers usually feel a strong bond with their baby. They want to hold the baby and have the baby with them after birth, even if they are tired or mother needs to be given medication. It may also be possible to have the baby stay with the parents even after a Caesarean, if there are no medical complications.

Some babies will want to nurse immediately after delivery. Others will begin some hours later. If you are very attentive to your baby, you will hear him making a natural sound very similar to the "Eh Eh" sound in Infant Speak before actually beginning to cry when he is hungry. We encourage you to respond quickly with bottle or breast to this sound, answering it in kind with "Eh Eh. Ma Ma is here," while beginning to feed the baby.

In this way, the baby will learn that his needs can be met through the use of words rather than by crying, screaming, getting red in the face, sweating, and raising his blood pressure.

Many hospitals require the baby be initially taken to the nursery for routine processing. Rooming with your baby has become common practice at most hospitals. To help baby feel safe and secure throughout the hospital stay, we recommend that he or she stay with mother.

Find out ahead of time what the rules are at the hospital where you are delivering your baby so you will know what to expect and can plan your interaction with your baby.

## How to Hold Your Newborn Baby

Because baby must be routinely examined by hospital staff during the first few days after birth, we recommend that the father, helper, and the mother learn how to hold a newborn safely and securely. That way, Daddy or your helper can take the baby to where he or she will be measured and weighed, stay with the baby and then bring the baby back to you as soon as the nurse or doctor is finished with procedures. Daddy's voice will comfort your baby during the examination.

Remember, your voices are the only familiar auditory stimuli your baby has at this time. This is the time to use your best soothing and comforting voice and hold the baby again as soon as possible after the examination so he can hear you as well as feel you.

Newborns need warmth – that is why they are always in blankets. Wrap your baby's blanket around him before you pick him up. That way he won't get cold and start to complain. However, once you take your baby home, you can also provide this warmth by having baby's skin next to yours and a blanket over the both of you. (Which would you prefer, a nice, warm body next to yours or being wrapped up in a cloth?)

It is best to hold a newborn by reaching behind her head and holding her neck and the back of the head in your hand, with your arm supporting her back in what is sometimes called the "football hold." Babies' heads are large in proportion to their bodies and tend to loll about until they develop better muscle control, so you want her neck to be secure and protected. When you pick up your baby, continue to breathe naturally and easily; this will increase your confidence. Move around a bit with some rhythmical motions. Make eye contact and let her hear your voice. Say "Hi *baby, this is* Da Da. *Da Da pick you up.*" Occasionally remind the baby about some of the exercises you practiced in the womb. If you used a special womb song or melody, this is the time to reintroduce it. Watch to see if your baby seems to recognize it.

Soon you will both be naturals at picking up your newborn. If you have friends with small children, you can practice holding your friends' infants before you have your own baby. Ask them to show you how they hold their babies, and what experiences they had in the first few days of caring for a newborn.

## Your Newborn

In the hospital, or soon after birth, you will be able to see that your baby will want to look at you and will feel comfortable lying on your breast and stomach.

At this time it is not necessary to use a lot of stimulation exercises. When you feel like it, try a few Primary Word exercises you used during pregnancy, but most importantly, enjoy the first few hours with your baby. It is a special time of bonding when your baby recognizes you from your voice and now can see what you look like.

Babies who have had prenatal stimulation may be more in control of their movements. They may also be able to perform tasks earlier than standard development would dictate. You may be able to maintain your baby's interest and attention longer. Because you have been talking to your baby for several months before birth, you and the hospital staff will find him or her very alert and responsive within the first few minutes after birth. You will expect your baby to listen to you.

Reassure him or her about sounds, actions, or procedures. On the first day of class, there is always a tendency for teachers to focus their efforts on children that appear to be "good students" and to expect more of them.

Fathers are often amazed when their babies seem to pay attention to their voice or turn their eyes toward father. We have had many reports of this occurring in prenatally stimulated babies shortly after birth.

## Post-Birth Stimulation

After the birth of your baby, we recommend that you begin infant stimulation as soon as you are reasonably able. Don't wait for a few weeks or a month when the baby *"seems to know what's going on,"* as one grandmother who was not familiar with Prenatal Classroom advised her daughter.

*Dr. Franz Baumann, who was a colleague and a friend of the family as well as our pediatrician, came to the hospital to make the newborn neurological examination the day after the birth of our first child. He was close to retirement and had seen thousands of parents and infants. He didn't know about the prenatal stimulation – singing and talking to our baby – that we had done during the prenatal period. He told us, "I say this to all new parents and some believe me. You ought to be careful what you say around that new baby of yours. After all, we never know when they start to listen." When we told him about the prenatal stimulation we had been doing during the months of the pregnancy, we all had a good laugh.*

(Comment from Dr. Lehrer on the birth of his first child)

Be persistent in the regularity of your stimulation exercises, but don't push the process when your infant is tired or irritable. Maintain contact with your infant and talk to him or her as if he or she can understand. Continue to talk to your baby and play music in the ways you have practiced throughout your pregnancy and hospital stay. For an awake baby, every family activity is a stimulating learning experience if you explain each thing to him or her as you are doing it.

You will find that a great number of routine "new baby" activities that are concerned with the care of your newborn can be used with our program.

## Feeding

You can begin infant stimulation with the baby as soon as mother has developed a sense of the baby's regular feeding patterns. Feed the baby for a little while so that hunger is satisfied but not so much that baby falls asleep.

While baby is in this semi-satisfied state, we begin connecting words he or she listened to during pregnancy with objects and actions they represent. For example, you can say, *"This is your nose"* (touch baby's nose), *"This is Ma Ma's nose"* (touch your nose), *"This is your mouth"* (touch baby's mouth), *"This is Ma Ma's mouth"* (touch your mouth), etc.

Touch your hand to baby's body part, then touch the same part on your body, then place baby's hand to his or her nose, then to your nose, etc. These intimate communication games are best accomplished during pauses in feeding rather than when the baby is actively sucking.

The side of the brain that controls language (Broca's area) is most likely to develop on the left side of the brain. However, recent research shows that boys tend to process verbal information in the back part of the left cerebral hemisphere. Girls' verbal skills seem to originate in the front part of the left cerebral hemisphere.

This same side of the brain controls the right hand. First touch baby's right hand and say, *"This is baby's right hand."* Then do the same with the left hand, so the baby may associate the actions and words in both sides of the brain. We believe this begins the process of developing good association pathways between the left and right sides of the brain.

Practice this with other paired parts of the baby's body, such as feet and ears.

## Words

If you have not used our prenatal stimulation program before your baby was born, you can start after birth with the Primary Word List and gradually incorporate words on the Secondary Word List while demonstrating to your baby what they mean.

The words you choose should focus on objects and actions with which the baby will become most familiar. These may include: feeding, eating, mouth, breast, nipple, crib, and the rooms of the house where baby spends most of his or her time.

## Scheduling Sessions

It may be difficult at first to schedule stimulation sessions for baby's wake time. If the baby is drowsy, you can wake him or her by massaging the soles of one or both feet. This will stimulate one of the "wake up" parts of the brain.

Can you stimulate your baby while he or she is asleep? Yes, the "position sensing" centers in baby's brain can be stimulated by rocking or motion. We can demonstrate the sleeping baby's skill in being aware of motion by the speed with which he or she wakes up when you stop rocking. If the sleeping baby awakens or becomes more active when the rocking stops, we know the baby had perceived the rocking sensation. If the baby is tired and doesn't easily wake up, wait until a little later when he is more rested and ready to be stimulated.

## Knowing When Baby Is Alert

It is best to have your stimulation sessions when your baby is alert. Here are some signs that your baby is ready to pay attention:

**1)** His or her breathing will be slow and regular.

**2)** The pupils of the eyes will be wide.

**3)** He or she will not be fussy, squirming around, or irritable.

**4)** During feedings, he or she may be sucking slowly or not at all. The cheeks will seem to soften because the muscles are relaxed and eyebrows are slightly raised.

**5)** The baby's head may turn to face you.

**6)** He or she will look at something held in your hand about a foot away, and the eyes will fixate on it. By this, we mean the baby's eyes will remain looking toward what you have in your hand instead of rolling around as he or she looks at other objects.

**7)** You may notice the baby's fingers or toes reach out in the direction of whatever has his or her attention.

At first you may notice that the baby has not yet learned to move his arms separately from his legs or one hand without the other. For an infant, moving an arm towards an object is in some ways the same as if you tried to pat your head and rub your stomach at the same time.

## Remembering Birth

The days you spend in the hospital after birth are also a good time to jot down a few notes about the birthing process and the delivery room. You and your mate should write down a few of the colors and objects you can remember that the baby might have seen as he or she was being born.

You can use these notes for your own reference in a couple of years. Or you may be interested in doing your own personal research on what babies remember. In that case, you might decide to ask your child how much he recalls about his own birth. Studies have shown very young children do remember this dramatic experience.

To be certain your child's answers are strictly his own memories, neither parent nor other relative should previously discuss the child's birth with or in front of him. You can pose the question to your child when he is about 2 or 3 years old. By that age he is old enough to verbalize complex thoughts. You may want to record this conversation for a keepsake. Or give it to your child when he is grown and ready to have his own children.

Here is the birth memory of a two-year old Prenatal University graduate as told by his father. The father was giving his son a bath at the time. For the first time, the boy was actively and persistently asking his father questions on a variety of subjects, which the father answered. Then the father decided to ask a subject of his own:

**Father:** *Do you remember being born?*

**Son:** *Yeah.*

**Father:** (noticing the faint sound of his son grinding his teeth) *What was it like?*

**Son:** *It was dark. A monster grabbed me and pulled me into kind of like a store.*

**Father:** *Like a store?*

**Son:** *Lots of bright lights and lots of people.*

**Father:** *What did the monster look like?*

**Son:** *He was green on the bottom and blue on the top.*

**Father:** *What did the monster do?* .

**Son:** *He choked me!*

**Father:** *You mean he grabbed you by the neck?*

**Son:** *Not by the neck, in the mouth.*

The boy had been born by Caesarean section at an urban hospital where the physicians and nurses wore green scrub suits and blue caps and masks in the operating room. After the delivery, the baby was placed on a warmer table, and a small rubber tube was inserted into his mouth and down his throat to remove any secretions that could block breathing. This produces a sensation of gagging or choking, the memory of which may have caused him to grind his teeth. His father reports that the boy was capable of accurately identifying the colors blue and green at the time of their conversation, and had never heard any details of his birth before he related this memory to his father.

That the boy perceived the obstetrician who delivered him as a monster is easy to understand. The doctor appeared immense to the tiny infant, he hovered around the baby, and the strange mask and cap in conjunction with the bright lights were frightening.

Birth experiences will be different for each baby. Perhaps due in part to the years of work by the Prenatal Classroom program staff and participants, hospital staffs have come a long way in the last few years trying to make birth as joyous an event for the baby as it is for the parents. Birthing suites that look more like home have replaced sterile delivery rooms in many areas. Physicians and nurses are more responsive to parents' special requests during the birthing process. We are pleased with the results, because everyone benefits.

However, whether or not your baby can remember his or her birth is not really the issue here. We like to think that some part of your child's brain retains a memory of the birth experience. Since the evidence seems to indicate that this is so, try to make the experience as pleasing as possible for your newborn. You can create a less frightening experience through the stimulation exercises you have learned.

## Going Home

Continue talking to your baby and playing music throughout your hospital stay in the same ways you have practiced for the last several months. If you have been using music in the hospital, play the same music you used during the delivery on the car stereo or on a portable cassette player when you take baby home. (Remember, most hospitals insist that you place your newborn in an infant car seat before you can drive her home). Playing familiar music on the way home will reassure baby about yet another new and strange event that is taking place in his or her life.

When you arrive home, you will be ready to start the next stage of using all you have practiced and learned with your wonderful baby.

Some parents report feeling self-conscious talking and explaining things to the baby on the street or in a grocery store. If you feel this way, you might try adopting the attitude of the mother who breastfeeds her baby in public. She believes this to be natural interaction between herself and the baby that is really nobody else's business. Our exercises are a kind of "mental feeding" that can continue until your child is old enough to explore and ask questions for himself or herself.

# Insights

## How Your Baby Thinks

Infants and young children perceive themselves as the center of the universe. They have no concept that other people think or feel any differently than they do. Their needs are all-important.

At some point in his or her development, your baby will assume mother feels exactly the way he or she does. The baby identifies so closely with mother that he thinks of himself as part of her, as baby, in fact, was during pregnancy.

Later, the baby will begin the process of venturing out from mother and becoming more independent. This process is called *separation-individuation* and has been found to be stimulated and enhanced by the following:

**a)** a close, strong relationship with the father in addition to the usual bonds with mother.

**b)** the infant's own high level of confidence and feeling of personal satisfaction.

At first, it may seem strange to think of your baby as a confident, personally satisfied, social person. Once parents start to think of their baby in this way, however, baby will be stimulated to develop along the lines of these expectations. We want babies to generate an internal feeling of confidence and capability with their world. We want them to function to the best of their ability and be aware that they are doing so.

Baby's confidence can be increased by parents who provide a loving environment. Parents should offer verbal support (*"That's good,"* *"Well done."*) as well as physical demonstration of approval (applause, hugs, kisses) when simple goal tasks are achieved.

We do not go along with unrealistic goals such as having the baby potty trained by one year, or insisting a toddler pronounce the word *"bottle"* correctly at the expense of his or her self-confidence and natural tendency for explorative behavior.

Parents who wish to conduct infant stimulation after birth can utilize the normal items in baby's environment. Baby can learn to touch, taste, smell, hear, and see the marvelous everyday items that you have come to take for granted. They are all new to baby.

Try to have at least two 15-minute stimulation sessions with baby each day. You should allow at least one sleep period between sessions to let the lessons sink in during sleep.

In general, we suggest that a stimulus be continued until it becomes apparent that is has been learned, but stop before the baby loses interest or the baby avoids it when it is presented.

Here is a chart that can help you structure your newborn's stimulation sessions:

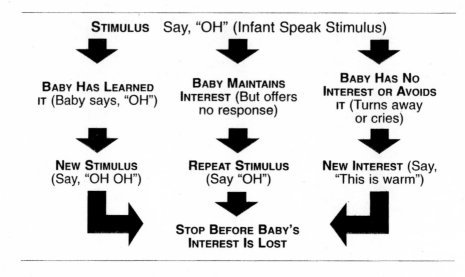

**STIMULUS** Say, "OH" (Infant Speak Stimulus)

| **BABY HAS LEARNED IT** (Baby says, "OH") | **BABY MAINTAINS INTEREST** (But offers no response) | **BABY HAS NO INTEREST OR AVOIDS IT** (Turns away or cries) |

**NEW STIMULUS** (Say, "OH OH")  **REPEAT STIMULUS** (Say "OH")  **NEW INTEREST** (Say, "This is warm")

**STOP BEFORE BABY'S INTEREST IS LOST**

## Introducing Baby to the World

After a while, you will know when your baby is satisfied, wide-eyed, attentive, and comfortable from a partial feeding. This is when you want to introduce objects to baby's world by letting him or her touch and hold them.

Start with the things that baby uses most, letting baby touch each object as you talk about it. For example, you can begin with, "This is your bassinet (crib, bed). This is where you sleep. This is your mattress. This is how it feels." Or, you can say, "Here is your blanket. This is how it feels." (place the blanket in baby's right hand and then left hand), "This is how it smells." (hold the cloth near baby's nose).

When you are putting powder on your baby, you can explain what you are doing and even why you are doing it. While you are carrying the baby from one part of your apartment or house to another, you can describe some parts of the trip to your baby.

You, as parents, need to include discussions with your baby in your daily activity. In that way, you will learn to spend quality time with your child despite a busy schedule. It doesn't really matter what your newborn understands. You are developing a relationship in which you are explaining things in your shared surroundings that are interesting and important to both of you.

During the first few days after baby arrives home from the hospital, try to familiarize him or her with the nursery. Help your baby touch objects first with the right hand and then with the left hand, holding the baby at arm's length from the objects and naming things as you go.

At very young ages, the baby quickly takes in everything but can't pay attention for very long. If the baby cries, fusses, or starts to hiccup, stop the exercise. That's enough orientation. The baby has reached his or her limit for now. Finish feeding baby and put him down for a nap.

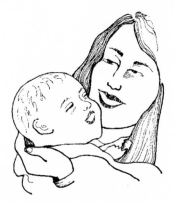

Each time baby wakes, it is like a new day, and the next lesson can begin. Introduce your baby to a new area each week. Start with the bassinet, then go to the bedroom, bathroom, rest of the house or apartment, garden, back yard, car, etc.

## Teaching the Concept of Choice

By six weeks, the baby is ready for the idea of choice. If you are bottle feeding, you might try preparing two formula bottles, one warm and the other cool. Then say, "Do you want a warm Ba Ba or a cold Ba Ba?" When you say "warm Ba Ba," touch baby's hand to the warm bottle, likewise with the "cold Ba Ba." And while offering baby a choice of breast when breastfeeding may depend more on which side the baby fed from last, you can offer baby a choice of which cheek he or she would like to place against you or what position he or she prefers for feeding. Either way, watch the baby closely for any motion, facial movement, or sign of preference. Be patient, repeat your question several times, clearly and slowly. Try to notice and pay attention to even the most subtle responses or sounds that your baby makes at these times.

When your infant begins to eat solid foods, other opportunities for decisions arise: "Do you want cereal or banana? Milk or apple juice? Water or milk?" When baby makes a choice, let that choice remain in effect until the baby tires of it. For example, if an apple juice bottle is chosen, don't take it away until baby indicates that he or she is no longer interested.

Do not worry about spoiling the baby by giving him or her a choice. You are stimulating those areas of the brain responsible for choosing and for decision making.

It is also important to realize that each baby develops at his own rate and expresses himself in his own way. Some babies are "active" and some are "observers." Your "observer" baby still takes in as much information as an "active" baby, but may prefer not to make as many choices or physical movements at this stage in life. For a more detailed discussion on this aspect of your child's development, see T. Barry Brazelton's wonderful book, *Infants and Mothers.*

You may not believe your baby is capable of the complicated thought process required to make a choice between two objects. It's not easy breaking through our preconceptions about the abilities of infants, especially those that have been passed down through the generations. However, parents who have participated in Prenatal Classroom have shared amazing stories with Dr. Van de Carr about the advanced abilities of their infants and their own heightened expectations.

*I was sitting on the carpet with my 4 month old son who had taken the Prenatal Classroom during his mother's pregnancy. Having been assigned the task of taking care of the baby while my wife was at the store, I sat near him, listening to his babble. He had become quite verbal and said some of the words on the Infant Speak List. He started to fuss, so I picked him up. His diaper seemed dry, but he continued to be irritable. I asked him, "Do you want a diaper change or a Ba Ba?" There was no answer, so I asked two more times. Then he said, "No, Dja De, Ni Ni." I put him into bed, and he immediately went to sleep.*

(Comment from a Prenatal Classroom father. The baby's word for Da Da was Dja De.)

This story demonstrates that babies can make choices much earlier than thought possible. Not only was the baby capable of making a choice, but he was also able to supply his own choice when neither the diaper change nor the bottle offered by his father were what he wanted.

People who don't believe babies can make choices may have never given infants the *opportunity* to make a choice. Instead, the adults have made the choices *for* their infants. We're not saying children should be given their way in every situation, but the practice of making decisions grows slowly through the making of small choices.

Our research has shown that babies can make choices at surprisingly young ages. Babies' lack of verbal skills leads many to believe that they have no preference. Babies aren't *expected* to make a choice. That is why Infant Speak is so important. These are words even very young babies can pronounce and use to explain their needs. Once you have given your baby these language tools, you too may be surprised at how complex his thought processes are and how perceptive he is about the world around him.

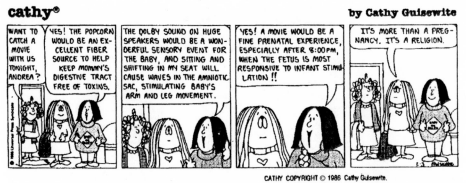

## Summary

The ultimate goal of the Prenatal Classroom is to produce changes in preborns and infants which will allow them to better deal with their environment and thereby live happier and more productive lives.

These changes in capability, sociability, and general awareness, when multiplied by ever-increasing numbers of youngsters exhibiting these benefits, will over time alter the fabric of our social structure.

If we can teach the infant to express his emotions, including: frustration and anger, through verbal communication rather than through emotional outbursts such as crying and screaming, we have altered the classic pattern of interrelating between mother and baby. So, instead of crying when he is hungry, baby will use the Infant Speak word "E*h* E*h*," and mother will respond, "E*h* E*h*," as she is fixing his bottle. Baby knows he will soon be eating. His need will be met without distress on his or his mother's part.

The most important basic principle upon which this book is based is that interaction between the baby and its environment stimulates brain growth both before and after birth. There is a critical time in an infant's development beginning at about five months into pregnancy and extending to about two years of life. During this time, neural interconnections are being formed in immense numbers in your child's brain. This is a window of opportunity to increase the number of connections through stimulation. You can increase your child's mental capabilities and ability to adapt to his surroundings by understanding and using principles presented by the Prenatal Classroom.

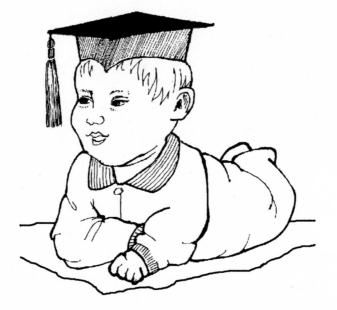

Furthermore, the Prenatal Classroom can help you become a more affectionate, responsive, relaxed, and emotionally nurturing parent, which is one of the major factors in the enhancement of your baby's abilities. The program provides you with a forum to get to know, understand, and teach your baby before and after birth in a loving environment that will set the tone for the rest of his or her life.

Thus, we see that the early relationship between the preborn baby and his or her parents has a profound effect on both the individual and society at large.

As a parent-teacher in the Prenatal Classroom, your training will help you to remain naturally enthusiastic, playful, and patient with your child for the rest of both of your lives.

## Always remember, the child who learns to like learning will learn.

# APPENDIX A

# The Prenatal Development Stages

| Weeks | How Your Baby Develops |
|-------|------------------------|
| 1 | End of your menstrual period |
| 2 | Conception occurs |
| 3 | Developing cells vibrate to your heartbeat (beginning now and continuing throughout pregnancy) |
| 4 | You realized you missed your period! |
| 5 | Your baby is large enough to be visible |
| 6 | Brain and major organs start to form |
| 7 | Eyes form (no eyelids yet) and muscles develop |
| 8 | Ear structures form |
| 9 | Your baby begins to make small movements, but you can't feel them yet |
| 10 | Your baby's heartbeat begins to develop |
| 12 | Your baby's toes and fingers form |
| 14 | The sex of your baby can be observed |
| 16 | Baby's eyes become sensitive to light |
| 17 | Mother can begin to feel occasional small movements |
| 18 | Baby's heartbeat can be detected, baby can now hear your heartbeat and other sounds |
| 24 | Baby has definite periods of sleep and wakefulness |
| 28 | Baby can "hiccup" |
| 32 | Internal organs mature |
| 36 | Kidneys mature and baby assumes final head down position |
| 39 | Lungs mature |
| 40 | Birth (plus or minus 1 week) |

# The Prenatal Classroom Program - Summary by Weeks

*Before Pregnancy:* Girl or Boy Diet, Good Health Guidelines, 7 Health Hints for a Good Pregnancy.

| Week | The Prenatal Classroom Program |
|------|-------------------------------|
| 1 | Environmental Do's and Don'ts |
| 2 | Accelerated Nutrition Before and During Pregnancy |
| 3 | Brain Growth Pregnancy Diet (up to 19th week) |
| 6 | Positive Visualization Exercises |
| 17 | Basic Drum Rhythms |
| 18 | Basic Growth Pregnancy Diet Part 2 (choline) |
| 20 | The Kick Game |
| 27 | Finding Baby's Position |
| 28 | Second Phase – Primary Words |
| 29 | Womb Stories, Womb Songs, and Womb Melodies |
| 30 | Building Pre-Awareness of Words |
| 31 | Third Phase – The Xylophone Game |
| 32 | Pre-Awareness of Numbers |
| 33 | Infant Speak |
| 34 | Secondary Words |
| 38 | Preparation for a "Baby-Oriented" Birth |
| 39 | Labor and Delivery Practice |
| 40 | Your Newborn at the Hospital |
| 41 | Your Newborn at Home, Insights Into How Your Baby Thinks |

# APPENDIX B

## Musical Selections

### Composers

**Bach:** The Brandenburg Concertos, any of the concertos for solo instruments and orchestra, the partitas, preludes and sonatas for various instruments, and the vocal/choral cantatas

**Handel:** The Royal Fireworks Music, The Water Music Suite, Messiah

**Pachelbel:** Canon

**Vivaldi:** The Four Seasons Concertos, any of the solo instrumental concertos

**Haydn:** The symphonies, concertos, string quartets, masses

**Mozart:** The symphonies, concertos, string quartets, Requiem

**Beethoven:** The symphonies, concertos, string quartets

### Specific Titles

Adagio Lucerne Festival of Strings
Airs from the Courts and Times of Henri IV and Louis XIII
Bach's After Midnight (*Denis Vaughan*)
Bach's Triumphs
Beethoven's Greatest Hits
Carnival of the Animals by Camille Saint-Seans
Chopin's Preludes
Lullaby from the Womb by Dr. Hajime Murooka (*includes recordings of heartbeat sounds from within the womb*)
Magical Strings (*Harp and Hammered Dulcimer*)
Nocturne by James Galway
Nutcracker Suite by Tchaikovsky
Pachelbel's Canon and Other Baroque Favorites
Pachelbel's Greatest Hits
Pictures at an Exhibition by Mussorgsky
Symphonic Bach (*Boston Pops*)
The Four Seasons by Vivaldi
The Planets by Holst (*all except the "Mars" passage*)

### Pop and Folk Music

The Marvelous Toy & Other Gallimaufry by Tom Paxton
The Folksinging of Burl Ives
The Folksinging of Tom Chapin
The Songs of Raffi

**Make your own:** Record a composite tape of selected favorites to play for your baby. You can also record a tape of mother, father, or other family members singing favorite songs to play for your baby, or for the babysitter to play in your absence.

# APPENDIX C

# Reference Material

Chamberlain, D. *Babies Remember Birth* (1st Ed.). New York: Ballantine Books, 1988.

"Does Diet Determine Sex?" *Parade Magazine*, p. 7, (Study by Joseph Stolkowski, Ph.D. from Pierre and Marie Curie University, Paris, France), June 27, 1982.

The Infant Health and Development Program "Enhancing the Outcomes of Low-Birth Weight, Premature Infants: a Multi-Site, Randomized Trial." *Journal of American Medical Association*, 263, pp. 3035-3042, 1990.

Logan, B. "Teaching the Unborn: Precept and Practice." *Pre- and Peri-Natal Psychology Journal*, 2, pp. 9-25, 1987.

Ludington-Hoe, S. *How to Have a Smarter Baby*. New York: Rawson Associates, 1985.

Panthuraamphorn, C. "The Effects of a Designed Prenatal Enrichment Program on Growth and Development of Thai Children." Thailand: Hua Chiew General Hospital, Poh Teck Tung Foundation, 1991.

Prescott, J.W. "Phylogenetic and Ontogenetic Aspects of Human Affectational Development." Presented at International Congress of Sexology, Montreal, Canada, 1976.

Rosenthal, R. and L.F. Jacobson. "Teacher Expectations for the Disadvantaged." *Scientific American*, 218 (4), pp. 19-23, 1968.

Rosenzweig, M.R., E.L. Bennett, and M.C. Diamond. "Brain Changes in Response to Experience." *Scientific American*, 226 (2), pp. 22-30, February 1972.

Smolan, R., P. Moffitt, and M. Naythons. *The Power to Heal: Ancient Arts & Modern Medicine* (1st Ed.). New York: Prentice Hall Press, 1990.

Ubell, "Lighten Up Winter Sadness." *Parade Magazine*, pp. 12-14, (Study from National Institute of Mental Health in Bethesda, Maryland, links mood and illumination, November 3, 1991.

Van de Carr, F.R. and M. Lehrer. "Enhancing Early Speech, Parental Bonding and Infant Physical Development Using Prenatal Intervention in Standard Obstetric Practice." *Pre-and Peri-Natal Psychology*, 1, pp. 20-30, 1986.

Van de Carr, F.R., M. Lehrer, and K. Van de Carr. "Prenatal University,"
*New Horizons in Learning*, 3, pp. 9-10, 1984 .

Van de Carr, F.R. and M. Lehrer. "Prenatal University; Commitment of
Fetal Bonding and the Strengthening of Family Unit as an Educational
Institution." *Pre- and Peri-Natal Psychology*, 1988.

Van de Carr, Kristin. "Effects of a Prenatal Intervention Program." *Prenatal
and Perinatal Psychology and Medicine: Encounter with the Unborn*. New Jersey:
The Parthenon Publishing Group, 1985.

# More Outstanding Early Learning Books from Humanics

*Teaching Terrific Twos* by Terry Lynne Graham, M.A., and Linda Camp. **$17.95**

*Teaching Terrific Twos* is a cornucopia of effective, mutually rewarding activities designed to keep that young mind as active as that toddling body. This wonderful guide to the fascinating mind of the two year old contains self-image, listening, language, social growth, movement, science, music, and even math activities designed for this special age group. Basic and individual learning goals are well-illustrated, from scheduling, materials, and teaching and learning techniques. A sample developmental skills checklist is included so you can assess your two year old's progress, identify weak areas, and reward strengths!

*The Infant and Toddler Handbook* by Dr. Kathyrn Castle. **$16.95**

*The Infant and Toddler Handbook* is a practical guide for parents, grandparents, teachers, caregivers – anyone who cares for and spends time with children from birth to 24 months. We all know how vitally important a child's first two years are to his or her social, emotional, physical, and intellectual development. *The Infant and Toddler Handbook* incorporates the latest in child development research into practical suggestions to use with your child anytime, in any setting. With these activities or "invitations," developmentally sequenced and arranged by area of development and age for easy use, you can be satisfied that you are doing your best to ensure your child's optimal social, cognitive, language, and physical development.

*Children Around the World* by Jane A. Hodges-Caballero, Ph.D. **$19.95**

What do people wear in Japan? What songs do people sing in Angola? What do people eat in Wales? Given the opportunity, no child is too young to begin to learn to appreciate the beauty and diversity of our world. Rich in resources for broadening the horizons of children from Pre-School to grade 5, Children Around the World contains descriptions, recipes, activities, stories, maps, flags, vocabulary and games from fifty-two countries throughout Asia, Africa, Europe, the Middle East, East Asia, South America, and the Caribbean. With this non-ethnocentric, entertaining activity book, you can help children recognize the subtle differences and universal similarities in people from vastly different cultures and settings.Help your children understand and respect the varied and unique cultures of our world.

*Toddlers Learn By Doing* by Rita Schrank. **$14.95**

These hundreds of activities will help parents, grandparents, other family members, and teacher stay ahead of a toddler's short attention span and boundless energy. You'll find activities for active and quiet play, stimulating the five senses, enhancing your child's language and concept development and fostering independence. You'll find new ways to use old favorites – sand play, water play, and playdough – and ideas for games, crafts, and cooking that use common, inexpensive materials. Give your toddler the broad base of experiences that is so important before preschool – positive, fun experiences that enhance your child's enthusiasm for learning right from the start.

*Fingerplays and Rhymes for Always and Sometimes* by Terry Lynne Graham, M.A. **$16.95**

Fingerplays and rhymes always delight children with their rhythm, imagery, and often humorous nonsense. Along with the fun, they can teach colors and numbers, develop finger dexterity and hand-eye coordination, and extend attention span. More than 250 rhymes and fingerplays deal with seasons, animals, feelings, self-concept, monsters, holidays, family, dinosaurs – all the topics that fascinate young children. Put these rhymes to work in your home or classroom and see how much fun (and learning) they bring!

*Birthdays: A Celebration!* by Marilyn Ateyo and Anna Uhde. **$14.95.**

This windfall for parents is packed with practical and exciting ideas for making children's birthdays into celebrations worthy of such an important event in your child's life. Here's how to stimulate children's creativity and social development as the whole family joins in planning, preparing, and enjoying these celebrations. No more stiff, boring parties! More than 30 party themes include Space Wars, Hawaiian Luau, April Fool's Backward Party, Teddy Bear Picnic, as well as a selection of Birthday celebration themes from around the world. More than 200 games and activities can be adapted for children of all ages. You'll find recipes for unusual party treats, directions for making invitations and decorations, and tips for cake-baking. The joy and memories of a truly wonderful party enrich your child's life – and *Birthdays: A Celebration* can make it happen!

*The Humanics National Infant-Toddler Assessment Handbook* by Dr. Jane A. Hodges-Cabellero and Dr. Derek Whordley. **$15.95**
(Specimen Set - Manual and 5 Forms - **$22.95**)

*The Humanics National Infant-Toddler Assessment Handbook* is the user's guide to the *Humanics National Child Assessment Form Age 0-3*, a developmental checklist of skills and behaviors which normally emerge during the birth to three year range. It also integrates critical concepts of child development into one system of observation and assessment. Designed for parents, teachers, and caregivers, this manual presents a comprehensive description of the effective assessment and specific activities to use to both assess and encourage your child's development.

**For more information on ordering these and other Humanics Early Learning materials, contact your local book distributor, book store, or call 1-800-874-8844 today!**

*Self-Esteem Activities: Giving Children From Birth to Six the Freedom to Grow* by Angie Rose, Ph.D. and Lynn Weiss, Ph.D. **$19.95**

Developed by two of the nation's foremost child development experts, these nurturing activities are arranged to parallel the five steps of a child's emotional development: trust, self-awareness, self-esteem, power, and self-control. An invaluable handbook of activities for parents and children (ages birth to six years). Remember: Children do not develop low Self-Esteem unless they learn it from others.

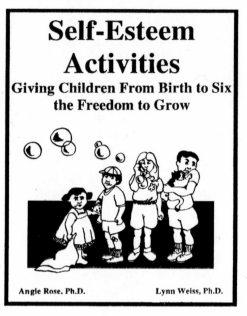

*Can Piaget Cook? Science Activities* by Mary Anne Christenberry, Ph.D. and Barbara C. Stevens, Ed.D. **$15.95**

This delightful book emphasizes the importance of food and the steps involved in the cooking process. These activities incorporate math and science skills that teach lessons about measurement and following directions. Finally, there's a way to mix food with learning! An innovative activity book with inexpensive materials – come and experiment in Piaget's kitchen.

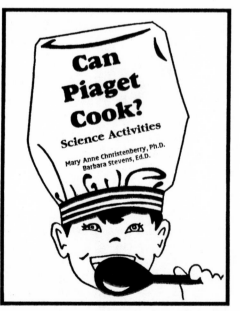

*Science Air & Space Activities: Folder Games for the Classroom*
by Jane A. Hodges-Caballero, Ph.D.
Adapted for preschool by Leah M. Hughes **$16.95**

"What do you wear on the moon? What do you eat in space?" These are but two of the intriguing questions addressed in this book, a "first of its kind" manual, that provides teachers, students, and space enthusiasts with a unique overview of aerospace education. Students will follow aerospace history from kites and balloons to helicopters, gliders, and airplanes through to today's satellites and the Space Shuttle.

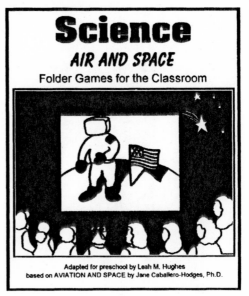

**Science**
**AIR AND SPACE**
Folder Games for the Classroom

Adapted for preschool by Leah M. Hughes
based on AVIATION AND SPACE by Jane Caballero-Hodges, Ph.D.

*Reading Resource Book: Parents & Beginning Reading* by Mary Jett-Simpson, Ph.D. **$19.95**

How to introduce children to reading, virtually from birth. Includes an overview of development, reading skills games, lists of resources, and an excellent section of book evaluations for young readers. Invaluable for teachers, parents, and other child-care providers.

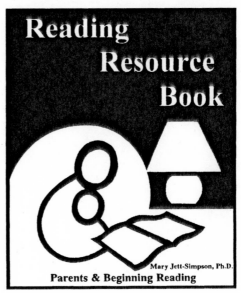

**Reading Resource Book**
Mary Jett-Simpson, Ph.D.
**Parents & Beginning Reading**

# About the Authors

F. Rene Van de Carr, M.D., F.I.C.S., F.A.C.O.G., holds patents for his educational, medical, and mechanical inventions which include the first computerized portable fetal/maternal monitor and the first infant respiration monitor. His work in the service of prenatal care and psychological bonding has made him a world-renowned pioneer in the field of early childhood education and development. Father of seven children, he lives in Central California with his wife Kristin, also a Ph.D., who works in the field of pre- and peri-natal psychology. Dr. Van de Carr is sought after as a speaker and trainer for prenatal development and stimulation.

Marc Lehrer, Ph.D., has been Staff Psychologist at the Child Study Unit in the Department of Pediatrics at The University of California Medical School and is a former President of the Northern California Society of Clinical Hypnosis. He became interested in prenatal stimulation when asked to consult with women experiencing stress during pregnancy. His stress-management methodologies and experience with prenatal stimulation form an integral basis for the Prenatal Classroom Program. He lives in Santa Cruz, California, with his wife Leslie and their two daughters Celene and Claire. Dr. Lehrer is currently conducting workshops at the Esalen Institute in Big Sur, California.

Printed in the United States
19559LVS00005B/385-387